Intermittent Fasting Mastery

(Complete Beginners Guide)

A Fast, Easy Plan For Rapid Weight & Fat Loss -
Including Spiritual Fasting, Prayer, Motivation,
Lifting, Affirmations, Success & Ketogenic Diet

Magnus Evans

Table of Contents

Intermittent Fasting

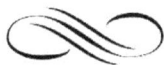

What Is It

You may have heard of intermittent fasting as being "The Diet" to lose weight and improve health. It's true!

It's an eating pattern that cycles between periods of eating and not eating (fasting). Unlike most diets, intermittent fasting focuses more on *when* you eat rather than *what* you eat.

If this sounds hard to you then think about this. You actually practice fasting everyday without even realizing it. When you're sleeping, you're fasting! Ever wonder why the first meal of the day is called breakfast (break-fast)? Doesn't seem that bad, now does it?

In the beginning, you may experience several hunger pains throughout the day, especially during your normal eating times. But over time, when your body gets used to not eating, those pains will go away.

You may be asking yourself, "If I'm feeling hungry and I don't eat, doesn't that mean I'm starving myself? Isn't starvation bad?"

This is actually one of the biggest misconceptions about fasting. It is not true! Starvation is involuntary whereas fasting is voluntary. You can start and stop whenever you feel like it. Although the key is consistency.

In fact, fasting is not so much a diet as it is an eating schedule. Thus, allowing you to get the most out of each meal. This is a particular problem with most people who don't absorb all the nutrients and healthy compounds in their food.

Fasting has been around for thousands of years and is revered as an ancient healing tradition. It has been known to improve concentration, prolong lifespan, increase weight loss and even reverse aging!

People all over the world fast for many reasons. In fact, every major religion in the world has periods of fasting. But whether it's for religious or personal reasons, there's no doubt that it will lead to a healthier life.

Natural periods of fasting have been around since the beginning of time. Humans and animals have always gone through cycles of low food availability. It's a completely natural process.

It is so ingrained in human history that our physiology has evolved to support this way of life. This results in a process of building, storing and eventually breaking down specific compounds in the body. Here is a rough breakdown of what happens during a fast.

During periods of eating the body raises insulin levels to increase glucose absorption for muscles and brain energy. Any excess glucose is stored in the liver as glycogen. Once fasting begins (around 6-24 hours after) insulin levels start to drop.

The stored glycogen then breaks down into glucose to release energy. This lasts around 24 hours. After 1-2 days of fasting the body goes through a process called gluconeogenesis. This is when the liver beings making its own glucose.

2-3 days after fasting the body enters into ketosis. Ketosis is a state wherein your body starts breaking down fat for energy. This produces compounds called glycerol, fatty acids and ketone bodies. The glycerol is used for gluconeogenesis, the fatty acids provide tissue energy and the ketone bodies give energy to the brain. During fasting, these ketone bodies increase significantly, over 70 fold. This is why many people report improved brain functions.

The last phase, which happens after 5 or more days of fasting, is protein conservation. Growth hormone levels increase to help maintain muscle mass and tissue. Basal metabolism is kept going by energy from fatty acids and ketones. Which in turn prevents a decrease in metabolic rate, contrary to popular belief.

There are several different forms of intermittent fasting that you can do, which will be discussed later on in this guide. Choosing one that best suits your needs and daily schedule is key to a smooth and effective start.

Why Should You Do It

If you want to try intermittent fasting to lose weight, then great! Studies have shown that intermittent fasting can help reduce body weight up to 7%. That's around a 12lb loss.

One specific study conducted at the University of Southern California had 71 people follow an intermittent fast for five days, every three months. On average they lost around 6lbs, reduced inflammation and slimmed their waistlines, all without losing muscle mass.

Besides losing weight, intermittent fasting also has other numerous health benefits. One in particular is improved brain function and lower risk of degenerative diseases. It has been shown to protect nerve cells from dying off and accelerate autophagy - a process that cleans out damaged neurons and grows new ones.

By lowering cholesterol, blood pressure and insulin resistance it has also been shown to help prevent diseases like cancer, diabetes and heart disease. Surprisingly, it can also slow down tumor growth in cancer patients. When done with chemotherapy, fasting can increase the levels of lymphocytes that attack the tumor, slowing and even reducing its growth.

Fasting is also essential for clearing out toxins that accumulate in your body from the air around you. Many people don't realize it, but your skin is actually one giant organ that absorbs everything that touches it.

This includes chemicals in lotion, shampoos, soaps, makeup and many other personal care products.

Our lungs also absorbs trillions of toxins from the air we breath. Even if you live in a rural area or somewhere surrounded by nature, their is still lots of pollution being put into the air from factories all over the world.

And lastly, our minds need a fast from all the information we are taking in at such a rapid pace. How many people do you know that are stressed from all the work they have to do, all the bills they have to pay and everything else that's weighing on their mind?

Taking the time to do an intermittent fast will not only help you get healthy and have the body you desire, it will clean out invisible toxins that are negatively affecting your body processes and your mind.

These are just a few of the healthy results you can obtain by fasting. The list goes on and on. You only need to try it out to begin seeing and feeling the improvements it has on your body and overall health.

Fasting is part of the natural way of life. It's no wonder it can cure many, if not all human health issues. By starting an intermittent fast you're putting yourself on the path to great health, a strong mind and ultimately, a happy life.

Beginning Your Fast

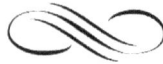

So you've decided to start your intermittent fast. Firstly, give yourself a pat on the back. Making the decision is the first step!

Starting something new is always a challenge, but by following this guide your beginnings into intermittent fasting will be easy. Not only that, you'll stick with it and soon be experiencing the amazing benefits that come with it.

In this chapter I'll explain the different types of intermittent fasts you can do, what type of person each one is suited to and how to begin your fast in a healthy way that will ensure commitment.

Types of Intermittent Fasting

In the fasting world there are 6 main fasting methods. Each one specifies different times in which you can eat and when you should be fasting.

It's important to think about your own habits and daily schedule when choosing which fast to do. Choosing one that is too complicated or that clashes with your daily routine can result in frustration and giving up. Simple ones that you can easily integrate into your life result in the best success.

16/8 Fast

This fast is the most popular and widely used, mainly because of its simplicity. The method involves fasting for 14-16 hours everyday and eating only during an 8-10 hour window. It's one of the easiest fasts because it generally only skips 1 traditional meal.

For example, if you eat dinner around 8pm then you're next meal would be around 12 noon. If you are person that needs breakfast then the opposite can be done. Your first meal can be at 8am and your last meal at 4pm.

During the time you are fasting, you may drink water, tea or coffee to help stay hydrated and reduce appetite.

This fast yields the highest success rate because it is the easiest to incorporate into a daily routine and therefore easier to stick to. It's ideal for people who are new to fasting and who have regular schedules.

5:2 Fast

The 5:2 fast is another popular one for beginners because rather than restricting eating times, you restrict calories.

For 5 days out of the week you eat normally. On the other 2 days you only eat around 500-600 calories each day. You can choose which 2 days to do this, but many find it easiest when they are not consecutive.

The appeal of this fast comes from its short spurts of fasting followed by extended periods of eating. It's best for people who are looking for flexibility and who don't want to completely restrict their eating just yet.

The Warrior Fast

The Warrior Fast is an intermediate fast and a good introduction into full day fasting. It was created to mimic the diets of ancient warriors.

During this fast you eat only small amounts of raw fruits and vegetables during the day. At night you eat one large meal. However, you can adapt this fast to your eating habits.

If you prefer breakfast then you can eat one large breakfast and only raw fruits and vegetables at night. The same goes for lunch, however it is easiest to adapt this fast to the beginning or end of your day.

Food choice is especially important for this fast, with a heavy emphasis on a paleo diet. Generally, you should be eating whole unprocessed foods that can be found in nature. If you're already following the paleo diet then this fast is tailored to you.

Eat-Stop-Eat

This fast is more advanced because it requires fasting for a full 24 hours. This should only be done once or twice a week.

You can fast from breakfast to breakfast, lunch to

lunch or dinner to dinner. If you eat breakfast at 8am on Monday morning then you'll fast until 8am on Tuesday morning. You are still allowed to drink water, coffee or tea during your fast, but you can't eat any solid foods.

On the days you do eat, it's important you eat the same amounts you normally do. This ensures weight loss and not nutritional loss.

Many people find this fast difficult to complete and it is not recommended for beginners. This fast is for someone who is comfortable with fasting and wants to take it to the next level.

Alternate Day Fast

This is another advanced 24 fast that requires alternating days between eating and fasting. There are 2 popular versions of this fast.

One version requires a complete restriction of food every other day. For example, on Monday you eat, Tuesday you fast, Wednesday you eat, Thursday you fast and so on.

The second version restricts your food intake to only 500 calories on fast days. On Monday eat normally, Tuesday eat 500 calories, Wednesday eat normally and so on. This fast is commonly known as "fasting mimicking" and can greatly increase weight loss.

This is a very challenging fast because it requires you to fast for 3 days out of the week. Many people report being very hungry on fast days leading them to binge on eating days. You should only attempt this fast if you are an experienced faster.

Fat Fasting

Fat fasting is essentially an advanced form of the ketogenic diet. It's a good option for people who are currently following the diet or for those who have hit a weight loss plateau.

This fast lasts for 2-4 consecutive days and restricts your caloric intake to 1000-1200. The key to this is that 80-90% of those calories are from fat only.

There is no eating or fasting time window, but some people choose to eat their calories in one meal, while others break it down into smaller meals throughout the day.

It's might not seem as hard as traditional fasting, but it has its own set of challenges. For one, food choice is limited. As most of your calories need to come from fat this leaves only a handful healthy options. Things like eggs, peanut butter or avocadoes are a great start.

Starting Safely

Once you've decided which fast fits you best, it's time to start incorporating it into your daily life. It may seem simple, straightforward and easy to start at any time, but it's better if you plan it out.

Easing yourself into a fast is the surest way to have a smooth transition, making it easier to stick with in the long run. It's also important to prepare yourself mentally and physically for a fast. Jumping into anything without the right preparation can not only cause frustration, but also harm.

During the start of your fast you're going to feel very hungry. Your body is not used to being deprived of food. The first few days, even weeks, of fasting will be the hardest as you get used to eating less.

Don't panic. This is very natural and not an indication of starvation. After about 2 weeks, your hunger pains should subside and you should start feeling more energetic.

To make the transition into your fast easy and safe, here are some things you should do before and during your fast. These apply to any of the fasting methods.

Consult a Doctor

If you're unsure whether you should fast or not, talk to a medical professional. Generally, most people can do a fast without it negatively affecting them.

However, getting a doctor's approval is never a bad thing. It is especially important for people with medical conditions. If you have diabetes, low blood sugar, are pregnant or trying to conceive, take medications or are underweight you should get a doctor's okay before starting.

Fasting with any of these conditions can lead to serious complications if not done properly.

When the doctor gives you the all clear or if you're healthy and well-nourished then proceed with the plan you've chosen.

Examine Your Current Diet

Part of fasting includes eating healthier foods.

You're not going to lose any weight if you keep eating junk food. You're also not going to feel very good if you binge on the days you can eat.

The key to fasting, losing weight and keeping the weight off is to eat healthy whole foods in moderate amounts.

It may even be enough to start your fast by simply eliminating any processed, high sugary foods you normally eat. When you begin your full fast this will help immensely with the cravings and hunger pains.

One simple way to eliminate bad foods is to substitute them with a healthy alternative. For instance, instead of eating chips you could eat some lightly salted nuts.

By filling your diet with healthy fats, proteins and complex carbs you'll feel less hungry and have more energy during your fast.

Start Slow

If it's your first time fasting take your time getting into the fast.

It's okay to have cheat days. It's even okay to spend a few weeks easing yourself into a fast.

Take this for example.

If you're doing the 16/8 method, but you get hungry during your 16 hour fast, eat a little snack. Don't do this every time you get hungry. But once and awhile, when the hunger gets to be too much, there's no shame in eating.

Remember to always listen to your body. It knows best.

Trying to power through hunger is the ultimate reason for failed fasts.

If it becomes unbearable or if you get light headed and dizzy, that's a clear sign you need some sustenance. That doesn't mean reaching for a pack of Oreos. It means eating a small salad or another light and healthy alternative.

Keep Hydrated

Chances are you're probably already dehydrated.

Many people drink far below the daily required amount of water. Not only does this cause numerous health problems, it also causes hunger.

That's right. Most of the time you feel hungry, you're actually just dehydrated.

By drinking lots of water throughout the day you can effectively reduce your hunger and appetite. It can also help with any headaches or dizziness you might experience.

Another option is to drink some caffeine. Black tea, herbal tea, coffee and sparkling water are tasty and keep you full. Just make sure they have zero-calories and have no sugar, artificial sweeteners included.

Plan Your Meals

Planning your meals for the days you do eat is an effective way to make sure you eat a balanced meal.

Many people struggle with controlling their hunger on the days they can eat. This leads to unhealthy habits like gorging. Stuffing yourself after a fast is unhealthy for your organs and can cause serious problems for digestion. It can also lead to weight gain.

By creating a meal plan you can be sure that you're getting the correct nutrition you need and the correct amount. It also forces you to stock your kitchen with only the essentials, lowering craving susceptibility.

Make sure to include your favorite foods into your meal plan.. Not only will this make fasting easier, it can be used as a reward for completing your fasting time.

If your favorite meal is considered unhealthy try to

modify it to include healthier ingredients.

It's also entirely possible to go out for a meal. There are plenty of restaurants that serve good quality, healthy foods. Just avoid foods high in salt, oil and sugar. Your stomach will thank you for it.

Stay Busy

Periods of downtime are when cravings and snacking are most intensified.

Think about when you're sitting in front of the TV or just browsing on your computer. You probably tend to reach for a bag of chips or some candy.

Staying busy can help with this significantly. Whether it's doing work or even exercising, by keeping your mind occupied you're less likely to think about food.

This means you should schedule your fasts so they coincide with times of the day/week that are your most busy.

Exercise is also a great distractor. Whenever you feel a craving coming on head to the gym or go out for a walk. Not only are you distracting yourself, you're getting out of the house and away from the kitchen.

Track Your Progress

The best way to see how intermittent fasting is working for you is by keeping a journal. Keep track of each day by writing down your thoughts and feelings. This way you'll be able to see how your emotions flow and prepare for days that you know are going to be tough.

If your goal is to lose weight, weigh yourself every other week and write it down. Seeing your progress will keep you motivated to keep going.

Taking before and after pictures is also a great way to see how you've changed. It's usually hard to notice any significant differences just by looking in the mirror. But taking a photo every two weeks or even just at the start and end will really surprise you!

Breaking Your Fast

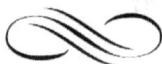

How you end your fast is just as important as how you start it. If not more so.

During a fast your body goes through significant changes. Your organs have adapted to having less food and have shrunk in the process. Your digestive processes have also been preserved to help you get the most out of the food you do consume.

What does that mean?

For starters, your metabolism has entered into a different state. It hasn't slowed (like many people believe), but it has started working differently. This affects your hormones and your physiology.

For instance, there is a significant increase in growth hormones and luteinizing hormones which produce testosterone. These hormones are great for building muscle mass and strength, but can be thrown off by sudden dietary changes.

If you were to break your fast by eating how you normally do, you would be putting a lot of stress on your gut. Not to mention possibly causing severe inflammation throughout your body.

There are certain things you should avoid and some

tips you can follow on how to break your fast safely and effectively. I'll be discussing them in this chapter.

What Not to Do

There are several things you should keep in mind when you're breaking your fast. The first is the types of food to eat and the second is when you should be eating them.

During a fast your body loses a lot of water. Along with that is sodium and potassium. Don't worry, this is not something bad. In fact, many people tend to have an excess, so think of this as a detox.

This does mean that you should refrain from eating high amounts of carbohydrates several days after your fast. Carbohydrates are antidiuretics which cause sodium and potassium retention in the body. This leads to bloating and a general feeling of sluggishness.

In general you should stay away from any heavy foods. This means anything processed as well as anything high in oil, sugar and salt.

But the food you really want to stay away from during the first few days after a fast is red meat. It takes a long time to digest and is therefore very hard on your stomach and intestines. It can also cause bloating and constipation.

When you do eat, avoid eating large meals. Overeating is a big problem for most when breaking a fast. It's also much worse when it's done following a fast than at other times.

This is due to the biological changes that happen during a fast. Normally, your body creates enzymes that help with digestion, but on a fast these enzymes are significantly reduced. Depending on how long you've been fasting for they could have been stopped completely.

The mucus lining of your stomach and intestines has also undergone changes. Daily production of it has stopped and therefore, it has thinned significantly. This makes it extremely vulnerable to inflammation. You should avoid eating anything that could cause irritation, like spicy foods.

What You Should Do

How you break your fast will depend on which type of fast you choose to do.

Breaking the 16/8 fast will be much easier and take less time than breaking the Alternate Day fast. But it is still important to follow these tips no matter which fast you're on.

First off, you start by only eating foods that are easy to digest and highly nutritious. This can range from fruit and vegetable juices to some simple soups or salads. Eating these foods in small amounts will help your body get adjusted to having food again and slowly start your digestive processes.

To give your digestion an extra boost you should

begin introducing live enzymes and healthy bacteria back into your system. This can be done by eating fermented foods and probiotics like sauerkraut and yogurt.

Just make sure to pay attention to your body. You may have a bad reaction to a perfectly healthy food, which means you're just not ready to eat it yet. This is why it's important to introduce new foods slowly back into your diet.

Watch for the feeling of being full. It's very easy to ignore when our bodies actually feel satisfied, leading us to stuff ourselves until we feel like we're bursting. Eating slowly will allow you to notice subtle changes and stop when your body feels nourished.

You make this easier on yourself by eating smaller meals more frequently. Every two hours for instance.

As a general rule you should only consume around 500 calories for your first meal. If you've been working out while fasting, this amount can be increased.

Work your way slowly towards eating more amounts less times per day.

However, if you prefer eating small amounts more frequently you can continue with that. You'll probably find that your eating habits have changed significantly since you started your fast.

One extremely beneficial thing you should do is to drink apple cider vinegar in the morning.

A tablespoon or 2 of this with water every day can really help your digestion. It stabilizes your blood sugar, balances out your pH and kills off any bad bacteria lingering in your gut. If the apple cider vinegar is too strong, you can also do this with freshly squeezed lemon juice.

Breaking your fast and returning to "normal eating" does mean your body will eventually return to burning glucose. But there are few things you can do to help keep it in ketosis.

One is to start the Ketogenic Diet, which I will talk about in a later chapter.

The other is to add some MCT oil to your meals. It stands for medium-chain triglyceride and helps with weight loss and energy. MCT's go straight to your bloodstream giving you energy faster, meaning you can continue burning fat and stay in ketosis even after you've eaten.

What To Eat

Now that you know how to safely break your fast, it's time to talk about what you should be eating.

I've said that you should avoid heavy processed foods and carbohydrates and that you should be eating nutritious easily digestible foods. So what does this leave you with?

A lot of things!

Here's a quick list of some healthy options.

Soft cooked veggies, raw fruit and vegetables, fermented vegetables like sauerkraut, avocados, yogurt, sprouts, eggs, nuts and seeds, soup, bone broth, beans and legumes and brown rice.

While all of these ingredients are healthy some are healthier than others.

For example, those that have been doing a 24 hour fast or longer should really be consuming bone or fish broth.

It's extremely important for your body because of the electrolytes and collagen it contains. It will also help you easily absorb minerals and electrolytes from other food as well.

Fruit is an interesting food on this list because it contains a lot of sugar that can only be metabolized by the liver. They're tasty and sweet which leads many people to believe they're a healthy snack or dessert alternative.

However, they do nothing to help your muscle glycogen. So if you eat fruit when you're already full the sugar gets stored as fat. They may be light and healthy but they will also take you out of ketosis.

You should really only be eating fruit as the first thing after a fast or after exercising.

When preparing your meals you will also want to begin by making them relatively bland. A few dashes of salt and pepper here and there won't hurt you. But don't add lots of spices or cover your meals with lots of sauce.

Adding fresh herbs is a good way to add some flavor without shocking your digestion. Plus, they all have numerous health benefits.

Working Out While Fasting

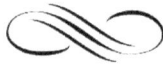

If you want to increase weight loss, tone your body and/or build extra muscle, working out while fasting is the best way to do that.

It's a common misconception that you should refrain from being active while fasting. This comes from the idea that your body needs to conserve energy while it is in "starvation mode."

But now you know that fasting is not starvation!

Therefore, working out and building or toning muscle is perfectly fine while fasting. In fact, many would say it's easier and faster.

The Ultimate Combination

By restricting your eating your body not only sheds it weight, it also goes through certain processes that make it easier for you to strengthen and build muscles mass.

The main process is the increase in fat and glycogen breakdown for longer and faster energy. This means you're not only shedding body weight, your losing overall body fat.

The reason many people, who don't fast, feel like

they're not losing weight even though they're working out is because of food. No, I don't mean eating a hamburger from McDonald's.

Even eating a healthy balanced meal before working out can severely inhibit your progress. This is due to the body's production of insulin.

When we eat, whatever we eat, insulin increases. When insulin increases, lipolysis is inhibited and lipolysis is what burns fat. So if you eat before a workout, you're only burning immediate energy from insulin while fat is still being stored in your body.

This also causes your muscles to experience oxidative stress which leads to muscle cramping and/or fatigue. But exercising while fasting prevents this by increasing acute oxidative stress.

Acute oxidative stress produces two compounds: glutathione and superoxide dismutase. These two compounds help your muscles increase their ability to use energy and fight fatigue. Letting you get the best out of every workout.

In a fasting state your body also produces more of the human growth hormone. This hormone in tandem with an increase in testosterone will raise your energy levels and increase your muscle mass.

In fact, the longer you workout and fast the more efficient your body becomes at burning fat. Even when you're not working out!

Most bodies today are not adapted to burning fat. They're adapted to burning sugar and sugar is not a good source of energy. It burns fast without offering much.

When you fast your body eventually gets rid of all those stored sugars and switches to fat. So when you exercise your body uses fat for energy instead.

By burning fat you'll be able to spend longer hours working out without getting fatigued.

Working out in a fasted state also causes the breakdown of intramyocellular lipids (IMCL) which is fat inside your muscle. You probably didn't even know your muscles contained fat.

When muscle fat is burned it causes an increase in the production of fatty acid binding proteins and uncoupling protein-3 content. You don't need to know what these are, just that they play a significant role in the growth and elasticity or your muscles.

Another amazing thing about the fasting and exercise combination is the body's increased ability to recycle and rejuvenate brain and muscle tissue. It's one of the reasons people find fasting to be an anti-aging mechanism.

Basically, fasting and working out keeps your body and muscles strong and healthy.

Getting your body to burn fat is key if you are an endurance athlete or simply have a goal of wanting to finish a marathon. Fat offers up an infinite amount of energy that will give you an advantage over all your competition.

Now I have to warn you, when you first start fasting you're going to notice a decrease in energy and exercise performance. You probably won't be able to run as long or lift as much. But this is only because your body is adapting to burning fat.

It must get rid of all the stored sugar first before it can learn to use fat.

Don't worry. This will only last around 2 weeks before your strength and endurance begin to recover. Soon enough you'll find you have more energy than you've ever had before.

So if you want to exercise go right ahead. Whether you're fasting for 16 hours, 24 hours or more, it is perfectly safe and even recommended to workout as you normally would.

Exercising Effectively

They type of workouts you should do depend entirely on what you want to achieve. Different workouts target different areas so it's important to narrow down your goal for better success.

If your ultimate goal is to lose weight and trim down on fatty areas then you should focus on cardio. Exercises like walking, running or biking are all very effective for this. But remember to vary your workout.

Lifting light weights or doing a few body exercises along with cardio is a great way to trim down and tone your body.

If you are looking to gain muscle and bulk up, you'll benefit from lifting heavier weights and doing workouts that focus on building muscle mass.

Further on, I'll talk about some different exercises you can do to achieve different results.

Choosing what time of day you exercise is also important. It's most effective when done first thing in the morning, before you've eaten anything. Eating before exercising can make you feel heavy and sluggish, leading to a poor workout. It's perfectly fine to eat a meal after your workout.

It's especially important that you eat 30 minutes after your workout if you've been doing heavy lifting. This is to give your muscles the proteins it needs to grow bigger.

Remember that everyone is different and it's important you listen to your body.

If you feel too hungry to exercise before eating then have a light meal before starting. Never exercise if you feel light headed or have low energy. You could potentially faint or get injured in the process.

Types of Exercise

From cardio, to weight lifting to yoga, there are many different types of workouts you can do. Each one has different regiments and does produces different results in your body.

They can all be done in combination with each other and in fact are very beneficial together. But if you have a specific workout goal, you should focus more on the one that will help you achieve it.

Cardio

For losing weight and body fat, cardio is the top option.

Cardio helps you burn calories, speeds up your metabolism and makes your heart and lungs stronger.

For an exercise to be considered cardio it must raise your heart rate, your breathing rate and challenge your cardiovascular system.

This means that leisurely activities, like walking, aren't really cardio exercise even though they're commonly thought to be.

In general, cardio consists of movement based exercises that are done for extended periods of time. This can include common workouts like running or swimming and even less common workouts like dancing and HIIT workouts.

Even everyday things, like gardening or moving furniture, can be considered cardio if done with the right intensity.

A good way to check if your workout is a cardio workout is with the Talk Test. If you find it difficult to say say anything, even small sentences, you're in a good cardio workout range.

So what kind of cardio exercises are there?

You have your standard everyday cardio. The ones the people know the most which include: running, cycling, climbing stairs and basically any cardio machine in the gym.

But there are also many other fun ways to get a good cardio exercise. This includes hiking kickboxing, playing a sport, dancing, martial arts, rowing, swimming lap, snowboard or skiing, and rock climbing, just to.

There are also many different versions of each that you can do. For example different sports include soccer, football or basketball and different dance styles include Zumba, Latin dance, breakdancing or even ballroom dance.

People find that martial arts is especially good because it offers a combination of cardio, strength training and learning self defense.

Either way, they're all extremely fun ways to exercise that you probably won't even think of as a workout.

Besides helping you lose weight, cardio workouts also have numerous benefits for your health.

Strengthening your cardiovascular system increases your lung capacity creating more oxygen flow throughout your body. In turn this helps bring blood to your muscles and clear toxins, such as carbon dioxide from your system.

Your resting heart rate also slows when your heart learns to pump blood more efficiently. This reduces stress on your vital organs by reducing blood pressure and helps prevent things like heart disease and strokes.

Mental illnesses, such as depression and anxiety can also be alleviated with cardio. During intense exercise, your body releases endorphins like serotonin and dopamine. These are natural pain killers that make you feel happy.

If you've never done cardio before, it's important to start slowly. Exercising for too long when you're not used to it can cause significant strain on your muscles causing injury.

Start out by doing only a few minutes of cardio a day at a low to moderate intensity. When you feel yourself getting stronger or having more energy, then increase both.

Ultimately, to get the most out of a cardio exercise you should be doing it for 30 minutes or more at least 3 days a week. The longer and more often you do it, the faster you'll see results.

Strength Training

Most people think of really buff bodybuilders when they think of strength training, but it's actually not the same at all.

Many men who do strength training do end up with large muscles like bodybuilders, however this is due to a specific workout regimen and an increased amount of testosterone.

Strength training is actually a great type of exercise for toning and building muscle.

Also known as weightlifting, it involves repetitively lifting different sized weights to strengthen and build muscle.

It's great way to lose weight and keep it off. In fact, if you lift weights 2-3 times per week for only 2 months you could lose up to 3.5 lbs of fat and gain 2 lbs of muscle. Not only that, for every pound of muscle you gain, you'll be able to burn 35-50 calories a day.

The scary thing is, if you don't work out your muscles with strength training they will eventually turn into fat as you age. It's a condition known as sarcopenia.

Strength training, however, doesn't just make your muscles stronger it also makes your bones stronger. This can help prevent degenerative diseases like osteoporosis. By increasing bone density, it can help prevent fractures and breaks later in life.

Injuries can also be prevented through the strengthening of connective tissues and joints. While this will make injury less likely it can also help improve recovery time if an injury does occur.

If your main goal is to lose weight, strength training is a fantastic exercise.

Studies have shown that lifting weights increases Type II muscle fibers which are responsible for improving metabolism. By building up these muscle fibers you could effectively eat higher fat and higher sugar foods without gaining weight. (Not that you should.)

If you play a sport or want to then you should be doing strength training exercises. It can improve your endurance, dexterity and hand-eye coordination putting you at the top of your game.

You'll also learn better posture.

Sitting at desks, hunched over computers all day puts enormous strain on your neck, spine and internal organs. Many health problems and everyday pains can be cured by simply correcting bad posture.

Strength training helps with that. It's actually extremely important for you to have the correct posture when lifting weights.

Bad posture will not only hinder your workout, it could lead to some serious injuries.

Lifting weights teaches you to stand straight and

engage your core during every exercise. This then gets translated into your everyday life. You'll be surprised how much easier doing everyday things becomes.

Your heart will also thank you for strength training.

Studies have shown that lifting weights dramatically increases blood flow within the body. In fact, after only 45 minutes of strength training exercise, blood pressure dropped by 20%. This is better than most blood pressure medication.

Improved blood flow was also found to continue for up to 30 minutes after the workout was finished. For those that lift several times a week for 30-45 minutes, this was extended up to 24 hours.

Strength training, like fasting, is great for your brain. It trains you to push yourself and go beyond what you think you can do. This is extremely beneficial for those suffering from mental illnesses, but it's also important for just dealing with everyday life. It's the key to success.

As with any exercise you should start slowly. Your muscles are probably not used to lifting heavy weights so you should start light. If you lift past your capacity you could end up tearing a muscle. Something very painful that takes a while to recover from.

Starting light also gives you the chance to practice good form, further reducing your chance of injury.

Begin with single sets and workup to multiple sets.

But remember to give yourself time to recover between each workout. 48 hours is the general recovery time between working out the same muscle group.

You should also switch up your routine to keep it from becoming monotonous. This means doing different exercises, changing the amount of reps or time between sets and varying your speed.

You'll keep your muscles guessing which will help with strength gains.

There are many different strength exercises you can choose from, such as bars, bands and free weights like the dumbells, deadlifts or kettleballs.

There are also many strength training machines like the leg press, the lat pull-down and the bicep/tricep bar.

And if you don't like using those you can even use your own weight by doing things like pushups, pull ups and situps.

It's important that you have a teacher with you if you are new to lifting weights. They will help you with your posture and ensure you don't strain or harm yourself.

By incorporating strength training into your workout routine you'll not only lose weight, you'll shave off any excess body fat you have and tone your muscles.

If you've ever wanted the perfect beach body, strength training will get you there.

Yoga

Yoga has been around for thousands of years. Today it is commonly thought of as a workout, but it is actually a system of philosophies, principles and practices used by Vedic Indians.

Yoga seeks to bring balance to the complexity of human nature by training the mind, body and spirit. This is done by combining focus on the breath with strength and stretching exercises.

It is one of the best exercises to do along with fasting because of its inherent philosophies. Through concentration, focus and movement you can bring calmness, centeredness and happiness into your life.

Unlike other forms of exercise, yoga is more than just physical exercise. The physical part is only 1 of the 8 different practices that yoga entails. However, for the purposes of this guide it will be the only part I talk about.

There are many different ways to do yoga and many different kinds of yoga.

The most popular forms of yoga today are Hatha, Bikram, Kundalini, Ashtanga, Vinyasa, Yin and Restorative yoga.

Hatha yoga is one of the original forms of yoga practice that is taught along with Hinduism.

Literally, hatha translates to force and is designed to

help one reach enlightenment. The practice consists of many different strength poses that aim to bring the right and left energy currents of your body to the center.

Different yoga teachers conduct different types of hatha classes. Some may be relatively easy and relaxing while others can be more challenging and strength focused.

Bikram is a form of Hatha yoga that is done in a heated room. It is usually heated to around 98-100°F (35-42°C) with 40% humidity.

The practice consists of doing a series of 26 poses for 90 minutes. The idea of this yoga style is to increase heat and sweat in the body. This helps loosen up joints and connective tissue to create more flexibility.

It also increases detox through the sweat glands. The poses practiced can be fairly advanced for a beginner as they require a lot of strength and movement.

Kundalini yoga is more of a meditative practice.

This yoga stems from the idea that our bodies a primal energy at the base of our spine. This energy, or kundalini, is used to wake up the chakras and help you gain enlightenment.

Kundalini yoga is deeply spiritual and focuses on movements that will awaken your kundalini energy. Although the class is mostly focused on meditation and chanting it has a physical aspect to it as well. Many poses must be held for several minutes, so the class does require a lot of stamina.

Ashtanga is one of the harder yoga classes and should only be done if you have been practicing yoga for a while.

The word ashtanga means eight limbs. These limbs include things like physical practice, breathing and pranayama. Classes are around 90 minutes long and should be done 6 days a week, if possible.

The practice consists of many strength and balance poses, twists and bends. The idea is to synchronize your breath with this poses to create an internal heat that will detox you.

Vinyasa is one of the most popular forms of yoga because of its versatility. It literally translates to "arranging things in a special way," which is exactly what you do with your body.

Like Ashtanga yoga, breath and movement are synchronized to bring balance to the body. But Vinyasa can be made easier or more difficult according to your ability.

It is very dynamic and the movements are always pre-planned to offer the smoothest flow between poses. You will probably break a sweat during this practice, but it won't be as difficult as some other yoga classes.

Yin yoga is a relatively new form of practice that focuses on holding poses for longer amounts of time.

The idea behind this form of yoga, is to get deep into

connective tissue and release any built up tension in your body. This means holding poses for 5 minutes or more. It is a slower class and the most passive out of all yoga classes.

All of the poses focus on flexibility rather than strength. Many people have a hard time with this practice because of discomfort felt from stretching for so long. However, once completed you will feel much more open and have a greater range of movement in your limbs.

Like Yin, Restorative yoga is also slower and focuses opening up the body with passive stretching. The idea is to learn how deeply relax all parts of your body which means very little movement.

This practice uses props to help ease tension out of your body while still allowing you to stretch your joints and connective tissues.

While this class may seem easy it is actually very challenging on the mind. Many people start to feel anxiety and agitation from having to be still for so long. But the purpose of this yoga is to calm your mind as well as your body and try to enter into a meditative state.

If you are new to the practice, then taking an introductory class would benefit you the most. Having an experienced teacher to guide you into the proper form and positions is important for getting the most out of your workout.

However, if you don't have time for a class or would

prefer doing it on your own, there are plenty of videos and apps with classes available online. These classes have excellent teachers that explain how to get into position and guide you smoothly through a flow.

A typical yoga class begins with an introduction consisting of some breathing and intention setting exercises that get you ready for your practice. This is followed by a light warm up, then a full flow and ends with some relaxing meditation.

Yoga is beneficial no matter how long or how often you do it. Even if you only manage to squeeze in a 10 minute practice once a week, you can still receive its benefits.

Many of these benefits include reduced stress, increased flexibility and strength, weight loss and improved athletic performance.

Increased flexibility is actually one of the main reasons many people start practicing yoga. Flexibility is extremely important for joint health and movement.

Yoga actually helps prevent joint and cartilage breakdown. By moving your body through its full range of motion you're essentially oiling them up. This can prevent degenerative disabilities like arthritis.

When you first start practicing yoga you'll probably notice a lot of resistance when trying to do the poses.

Your muscles and tendons have tightened over the years making you more rigid. Continuous yoga practice will loosen you up making it easier for you to move and giving you more range of movement.

Surprisingly many pains in your body are caused by something unrelated. For instance, tightness in the hamstrings can create poor posture and flatten the lumbar spine causing lower back pain.

Yoga will help aches and pains like this disappear. This is because it puts your body in proper alignment so that you are not straining any muscles or putting any extra pressure on specific parts of your body.

Mental problems like depression, insomnia and addiction can also be helped with yoga. This is because of the reduction in cortisol levels that occurs when you practice yoga.

Normally, when your body goes through intense periods of stress or trauma, cortisol is excreted through your adrenal glands. If this continues to happen it can lower your immune system making you susceptible to various illnesses.

These include mental illness. Excess cortisol in the brain can cause memory damage and permanently alter how you brain works.

But by lowering cortisol and teaching concentration problems such as these are usually cured with continued yogic practice.

Everyday Exercise

If you find it hard to make time to go to the gym or a workout class, then this special category of exercise might be for you.

It is not an official form of exercise, but it is one that can easily be adopted into your daily routine.

You may be surprised to find out that simple changes to your life can result in more activity and a daily workout.

Take going to work for example. You probably take a car to work, but you could easily switch to riding a bike and get in a good cardio workout twice a day. That is, if you don't have to go on any major highways.

You could even walk if you lived close enough.

If your work is too far and you have to use a car or if it's too dangerous to bike or walk then you can always just park your car further away. Adding that little bit of exercise to your daily routine can really add up in the long run.

Let's say you've been wanting to spruce up your house. Instead of calling someone to do the work for you, you could move the furniture by yourself or with a friend. Lifting couches and pushing bookcases is a great way to work out your arms and legs without you having to go to the gym to lift any weights.

Gardening can also be an intense workout if done for extended periods of time. Things like pulling weeds, lifting and potting plants and soil and rearranging pots can provide a good workout for your legs, back and arms.

Just make sure to not overwork your back. Continuous bending over and lifting of heavy objects can put a lot of strain on your back and even cause serious injury.

Cleaning is another activity that must be done routinely, so why not turn it into a workout? To get the most exercise out of cleaning combine several different activities into one day rather than spacing them out throughout the month.

For instance when you have time you can spend the day sweeping, mopping, dusting and wiping down windows. This will result in a good combination of cardio, strength training and even stretching. Plus at the end of the day you'll have a clean house!

Getting an active pet like a dog is also a great way to motivate you to get out of the house and to exercise. Generally dogs should be taken out two times a day which is ample amount of time for you to get in a good workout.

You can do many activities with your dog like going for walks, running and hiking. Not only are dogs great motivators they also provide you with company during your workout.

Lastly, if you've ever wanted to get more involved with your community or in non-profit help volunteering will allow you to do that and also provide you with exercise. Many places need volunteers to do physical labour such as lifting heavy things and running around to complete tasks.

It's a great way to get in shape and also give something back to the community.

Spiritual Fasting

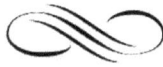

Along with all the healthy physical benefits of fasting comes the much less known area of spirituality and its benefits.

Cleansing your body also includes cleansing your mind and your soul.

Spirituality is a deeply personal thing and therefore it means different things to different people.

If you don't believe in anything spiritual, a spiritual fast could just mean a clearer mind and stronger motivation. For others it can be a gateway into cleansing spiritual blockages and reawakening life vigor.

Spiritual fasting can also help people deal with many negative emotions and difficult life situations. Things like a loved one passing, overcoming addiction, dealing with mental health or struggling to find a sense of purpose can be examined and dealt with in healthy ways.

If you are struggling with any of these things or simply feel some sort of blockage in your life, then a spiritual fast might just be for you.

What Is It

Essentially, a spiritual fast is a physical fasting.

Food is one of the body's most basic needs and by denying it that you can shift your focus inwards. Towards spirituality.

By starting a fast you're already putting your faith in something. Faith that your body will keep you going. Faith that you can control your urges and cravings. Faith that the fast will get you to your goal.

That's what spiritual fasting is at its core. It's learning to have faith and finding out where to focus it.

How many times have you turned to food when you've felt stressed or emotional?

This type of over eating is very common. Many people would rather try to pacify negative energy with food rather than deal with it. However, this inevitably leads to weight gain, emotional blockage, a buildup of negativity and an unhealthy relationship with food.

Fasting breaks this cycle.

Many people see fasting as denying yourself something you need. In reality it's actually learning to manage your needs so that you can work on other things that are more important.

As I mentioned before, spiritual fasting is something very personal. This means it will be different for everyone. It also means that it should be done for your own personal reasons and not as a way to show off.

In today's world everyone advertises everything they do. Diets and health trends are especially popular. So, when many people start a fast they also like to talk about it.

They use it to show off how strong willed they are or even how spiritual they are.

But spirituality requires humility. By all means, show off your physical progress, if that is one of your goals, and be open about your experience, but remember to be humble in your journey.

Refraining from making your fast public can also be seen as another type of fasting. A social media or technological fast. Taking a break from both can serve your mentality and spirituality immensely.

You may even find that you no longer have a desire to share as much.

Here are some changes that you can expect to go through when you complete a spiritual fast. Spiritual clarity, a cleansed soul, stronger or renewed faith, becoming in tune with the world and others and self empowerment.

Going through a fast with an aim of exploring spirituality allows you to increase your self-knowledge. In fact, one of the first things people discover is that they're stronger than they think.

On a deeper level, fasting also reminds you of the

spiritual connections you have to your physical body and where you stand in the world.

Fasting allows you to clear away all the debris of conditioning and artificiality. With a clean slate you can then start to see the beauty in the world and find your life's calling.

You'll also be able to clear out all the negativity in yourself.

People suffering from mental illnesses, like depression or anxiety, find this especially beneficial. By examining yourself inwardly you can see where these illnesses stem from and start to work through them.

Addictions can also be cured through spiritual fasting. By learning to ignore your body's most basic desire, you'll learn how to ignore short term desires, like smoking a cigarette. And you can take this lesson with you for a lifetime. You'll never fall back into your addiction again.

Once you've lightened the weight on your body and mind you can start to live more freely and happily. All that negativity has been cleared away, leaving enormous amounts of space to fill with love, enjoyment and positive energy.

With renewed physical and spiritual energy you'll be able to push yourself forward into the life you've always wanted. You'll find that you have more energy than you've ever had before, which you can use to explore and grow your faith/purpose.

Hildegard's Fast

I want to give a special mention to Hildegard of Bingen because of her research and devotion to the benefits of fasting and spirituality.

Hildegard was an extremely spiritual person born in 1098. Her life was dedicated to religion and holistic healing. She believed that illness could be cured through natural remedies and the balancing of mind, body and spirit.

She wrote many works on spirituality and became very famous. People would come from all over Europe to seek her advice on health and life. Many royal figures, and even the Pope, would write to her, asking for her words of wisdom.

Eventually she was made a Saint and today she stands for holistic teaching, finding harmony in ourselves and with all other creatures and the presence of the universe in every individual.

To achieve balance in the self, Hildegard believed fasting was the key. Because she was a nun, fasting was typical for her. But through this she was able to discover its true benefits which she could then pass onto others who were seeking help.

Her fasting program became known as Hildegard's fast.

It is an easy fasting program that slowly increases in difficulty without ever completely restricting food.

You are allowed to eat, but only specific foods and only in limited amounts. These foods must primarily consist of soup, fruits and vegetables.

You can choose to have days with no eating or days where you eat normally based on how your feeling. Hildegard's fast is not about starving yourself or even attaining any physical goals. It is about avoiding harmful foods that weaken your body and focusing your attention on your relationship with the spiritual.

In her writings she outlines 3 types of fasts which should be done in consecutive order.

Spelt Fast

This is the lightest fast out of the three. It includes a diet of spelt, vegetables and fruit. The spelt should be eaten in some form with every meal.

It is the easiest because it focuses on the overall benefits of eating healthy rather than restricting calories. It is a great introduction to taking a break from traditionally heavy eating habits and focusing on getting more nutrients.

The primary goal of this fast is to eliminate excess animal and milk protein as well as high fat foods.

You should be exercising regularly along with this fast. This helps promote the loss of toxins in the body and speeds of the fasting process.

Regular exercise is also recommended because you will be eating the same or possibly even more calories. Hildegard recommends at least 1 hour of exercise everyday while doing this fast.

A one day plan for this Spelt Fast looks like this.

Breakfast should consist of a bowl of spelt porridge with fruit and some spices. Some examples of this are raisins, apples, cinnamon, psyllium (dietary fiber) and even galangal (a spice from the ginger family).

Lunch according to Hildegard should be the biggest meal of the day. There are many options for this meal including spelt pizza, spelt pasta and spelt rice all cooked with a variety of different vegetables.

Lastly dinner should be a very light meal. It can include spelt porridge, spelt soup or spelt bread with simple vegetarian spreads.

Water should also be drunk throughout the day. However you can also drink fennel tea, coffee made from spelt, apple juice and even cut wine.

Cut wine is made by boiling a cup of white or red wine then adding a shot of cold water. The wine should be sipped on while it is still warm.

The Spelt Fast can be done for 6 months.

Bread Fast

This is the middle stage of fasting. Although it is an intermediate fast it is still very flexible.

It still excludes eating animal and milk protein as well as high-fat foods. But rather than changing your diet, it simply switches between the Spelt Fast and the Hildegard Fast.

When it is done properly it stops the feeling of hunger and even reduces appetite. This has the added benefit of weight loss. Because you aren't eating animal protein your body will start to breakdown fat for energy like in previous mentioned fasting methods.

A simple plan of this fast looks like this.

On day one you follow the dietary plan for the Spelt fast.

While on day two you follow the plan for the HIldegard fast, mentioned below.

For breakfast, eat a small bowl of spelt porridge with fruits and spices.

Lunch can either be a spelt salad, spelt rice, spelt porridge or a spelt semolina soup.

And finally dinner should be some spelt bread with fennel tea.

You should drink liquids daily and can consume the same things as in the Spelt Fast.

This fast can also last for 6 months.

Hildegard Fast

This is the most difficult of all three fasts, but is the

most spiritually rewarding.

You should give yourself 2-3 relief days to prepare yourself for this fast. This doesn't mean binge eating, but you may eat normal foods in a moderate amount.

To make the transition into this fast the easiest to to refrain from eating any animal protein or dairy.

The idea of this fast is to stop eating any solid foods for 6-10 days. The liquid foods are also restricted to a certain few. These include spelt coffee, fennel tea, spelt semolina soup, spelt soup and/or fresh fruit juice mixed with fennel tea.

A typical daily plan looks like this.

Breakfast consists of fennel tea or spelt coffee.

Lunch is a simple serving of spelt semolina soup with pureed vegetables.

And dinner can either be spelt soup, fruit juice with fennel tea or fennel tea.

Completion

When completing these fasts the traditional way to end them is with an apple baked in honey, cinnamon and sweet almonds.

Any food you eat afterwards should be chewed carefully and thoroughly to help ease your digestive process. Like any fast you should slowly reintegrate normal foods into your diet starting with the lightest and most easily digestible.

Refrain from eating meat, dairy and any calorie dense foods for the first week after your fast and pay close attention to your bowel movements. Typically you should be going 30 minutes after your meal but at a minimum you should be going at least every day.

If you are constipated take 1-3 teaspoons of psyllium before every meal.

A post fast plan should look something like this.

For breakfast eat either a small bowl of porridge with apples and spices or some spelt pancakes with fruit.

Lunch can consist of a salad with spelt grains, spelt pasta with vegetables or a spelt risotto.

And lastly dinner can either be a fennel salad, spelt casserole or spelt bread with vegetarian spreads.

Prayers

During the start and duration of your fast, spiritual connectivity can be furthered through prayer and meditation.

Many fasting practitioners, including Hildegard, recommend using prayer and meditation to help prepare yourself for a fast and to keep you going during it.

The basic idea is to set an intention every morning, something you want to work on, that you can focus on throughout your day. This will help with the hunger, but will also help move you forward spiritually.

If you are already a religious person then praying can help open doors within yourself and bring you closer to God. It is also a good time to confess your sins and rid yourself of any negativity and guilt that may be holding you back.

For those that are not as religious you can focus on meditation. Recognizing your faults and working through negative things that you want to change. This will bring you closer to yourself and help you open up to the world of possibility.

Whether it's through prayer or meditation acknowledging the faults we have in ourselves can help us focus on changing them during a fast.

It also opens you up to letting that negativity in your mind and spirit detox along with your body.

Often times people say they would meditate or pray more if they had the time. Fasting gives you that time, literally and figuratively.

By not having to spend so much time preparing food and eating it, you now have more time to devote yourself to exploring inwardly. This allows you to slow down and discover who you truly are and what you were meant to do.

You can also reflect on the things you've currently been doing. How much of those things do you like?

How much of it do you feel is actually you? If you could do anything in the world right now, what would you do? What's stopping you? These are things to think about.

There are two ways to practice spiritual fasting: meditation and prayer. I'll talk about both in this chapter and include some prayers/meditations to get you started.

Meditation and Fasting

Fasting is often done in tandem with yoga for serious yoga practitioners. This is because of the belief that it rids the body of tamas, otherwise known as darkness or negativity.

In yoga it is believed that everyone has tamasic elements and when they are out of balance it results in ignorance, dissatisfaction and materialism. Fasting helps balance out the tamas, leading to clarity and strength of mind.

This in turn helps with meditation.

Fasting helps create awareness and being aware of your body is one important factor for successful meditation and spiritual growth. If you aren't aware of yourself, good and bad, then how can you seek to fully change?

If you've never meditated before you may be asking, "Where do I begin?"

For starters, it's not just sitting on the floor for hours, trying not to think. Well, it is and it isn't.

Trying not to think isn't really the goal. The ultimate goal of meditation is to clear your mind. That may sound like I'm saying, "Don't think," but I'm not.

Clearing your mind means freeing yourself from distracting thoughts so that you can look at things from a different and more open perspective. Whether this is dealing with a problem you have or trying to overcome something negative, it's all the same.

Overthinking and distracted thinking keep you from finding real solutions to any problems you might have. You might say they're the toxins of the mind. Meditation is the spiritual fast.

The benefits of spiritual fasting are numerous.

A term has actually been created to label what happens from prolonged periods of meditation. It's called the "relaxation response."

This term refers to the many benefits that meditation has on the nervous system. Things like lowered blood pressure, improved blood circulation, lower heart rate, less anxiety, less depression, deeper relaxation and increased feelings of well being.

All of this can be achieve simply by setting aside a few minutes a day to practice meditation.

However, many practitioners say the goal of meditation is actually no goal. You simply learn to be present.

Buddhists say that the ultimate benefit of

meditation is the freedom from attachment. Particularly attachment to the things you can't control.

Often times we dwell on the past and things that went wrong. Regrets and guilt are heavy emotions to carry with you all the time but meditation can free you from those feelings.

You'll be surprised just how light you feel, once you've completed a meditation.

There are several different ways to meditate that are great introductions into the field. I'll talk about some of the more popular ones.

First off, let's talk about position. There are many different types of meditation poses, the two most common being sitting and lying down. Beginners often find lying down to be the easiest one to start with and then slowly progressing to sitting.

However, there are also active forms like walking meditation. Going on a simple stroll without a predetermined destination allows your mind to stop thinking for a while and relax.

No meditation is better than the other so just choose the one you feel most comfortable with. This will allow you to relax more and achieve a clearer mind faster.

If you don't feel like you can practice meditation on your own there are plenty of guided meditations available online that can help you through the process. Joining a yoga or meditation class is also another great option.

Here are three introductory types of meditation to help get you started.

Concentration Meditation

This type of meditation has you focus on a single point. This could mean following the breath, repeating a mantra, staring at a candle or listening to a repeating sound.

It may sound easy, but people tend to significantly lack the ability to focus on something for extended periods of time. You may find that you can only do concentration meditation for a few minutes.

You will probably get distracted during this meditation. Don't get frustrated or angry with yourself. It's natural.

If it happens simply return your focus to that single point.

Practicing this meditation daily or even weekly will drastically help you improve your concentration.

It will also help you learn to let things go. Rather than dwelling on a random thought and overthinking it, you'll simply release it.

Here is a concentration meditation exercise you can start practicing with.

First, find a quiet spot that is free from any

distractions.

Make sure you are wearing loose clothing that won't bunch or cut off any circulation.

Either sit or lie down, whichever is comfortable for you. You shouldn't experience any pain or discomfort during the entirety of your meditation.

Set a timer for 5 minutes, then slowly work your way up to meditating for longer periods of time. You'll be surprised how long 5 minutes actually feels when you're not doing anything.

Softly close your eyes and focus your attention on your breath. You can either focus on breathing in and out, on the time it takes you to do each one or on the number of breaths you take.

Whenever your mind starts to wander or becomes distracted by a thought simply bring your focus back to the breath.

Don't try to concentrate too hard on your breath, rather let your focus be light and natural.

Mindfulness Meditation

This type of meditation focuses on observing your thoughts.

Whenever a thought enters your mind you take note of it.

Rather than interacting with the thought or judging it, you simply watch it in passing.

Try to recognize what emotions arise in you when the thought comes without actually engaging with them. Are you stressed, angry, annoyed? Let those feelings and that thought go as easily as it came.

This is a very hard thing to do for many people, but extremely beneficial.

People tend to think in similar patterns that show up under the disguise of different thoughts. By being mindful of your thoughts you can soon recognize these patterns and slowly work to change them.

Through mindfulness meditation you will learn to find inner balance. This will help you become less quick to judgement and more accepting of things that are different than you.

Practice this simple mindfulness exercise everyday to ground yourself in the everyday.

Start by thinking of something that happens to you more than once everyday that you never really think about. It can be something as simple as a door opening.

Now whenever you touch a door or a doorknob pause for a moment and think about where you are. Where are you going? Where did you come from? How do you feel?

Take a moment to be thankful for all the things that allow you to be there in that moment. Be thankful for all the things that will happen once you walk through the door.

This practice is called a touch cue and can be down with anything in your life. The idea behind them is to bring awareness to everything in your life, even if it's the simplest thing. Rather than going through life on autopilot you learn to be thankful for every tiny detail.

Compassion Meditation

This is a unique type of meditation that many Buddhist monks practice daily. It involves learning to feel compassion for any and all things.

The idea of this meditation is to invite love and positive feelings into your body and soul which in turn will make you accepting and loving in your daily life.

Whenever a negative thought comes into your mind, try thinking of it in a positive light. If it's someone who wronged you think about what might have caused them to do this and try to forgive them.

This is especially beneficial for learning self-compassion. Typically, your harshest critic is yourself. But negative self talk can be extremely harmful for your mind and your spirit.

Compassion meditation is difficult for many because people are not prone to being forgiving. When something negative happens to us we tend to add more negativity on top of it. It's easier than trying to make it positive.

But practice makes perfect. Soon you'll be thinking and living more positively than you ever thought you could.

Here is an exercise in self compassion that you can practice whenever you feel a negative thought or emotion coming up.

One of the easiest ways to learn self kindness is by thinking of yourself as a good friend. You wouldn't tell your friend mean things or try to put them down, would you? No.

Think of your negative thought as something your friend said about themselves. What would you say to them? How would you comfort them?

Write it down.

Close your eyes. Take a slow deep breath. Open your eyes.

Now take a look at what you wrote and say those things to yourself.

Keep a list of all the positive things you write down and repeat them to yourself whenever you start to feel down. Positive affirmations like those can drastically change your mood and thinking.

Prayer and Fasting

Praying and fasting is an ancient tradition that goes

back as far as the oldest religion. In fact, every modern day religion advocates some form of fasting.

Christians practice Lent, which is a 40 day fast. The Jewish have Yom Kippur, a 25 hour fast of food and liquid (including water). Muslims have Ramadan, which is a fast of food, liquids and sinful behavior from dawn till sunset for 29 to 30 days.

They do this because they believe that the combination of prayer and fasting brings them closer and in deeper communication with their God.

There really is no difference between modern day fasting this type of fast except for the added element of prayer and the ultimate goal.

Modern day fasts are generally used to lose weight, get in better physical condition and heal many sicknesses. These benefits still happen for pray and fast, but they are not the goal.

The goal is to gain a deeper relationship with God.

The thought is that by taking focus off of physical things in the world (ie. food), a person can focus more on God.

Other things can be sought after as well with prayer and fasting such as humility, repentance, seeking God, asking for something, to know God's will and developing discipline.

If you haven't ever combined payer and fasting before you may be wondering how to do it and how often you should.

There aren't any hard set rules. It's all completely personal.

You can pray everyday, every week or whenever you feel like it. But most say the more often you pray, the better your connection to God.

Prayer can also be a private or public affair.

If you are part of a church you might want to pray with others. But you may also want to go into seclusion during your fast and pray in private.

The benefit of praying in seclusion is to minimize distractions and gain deeper introspection.

So how do you pray or how should you pray?

This is also up to your personal preferences.

There are plenty of prayers for you to call upon, but you may also prefer to create your own prayers. This way you can personalize your message and feel like you're connecting on a deeper level with God.

If you've never prayed before, here is a simple favorite that you may have heard before. It's called The Lord's Prayer.

Our Father, who art in heaven
Hallowed be thy name.
Thy kingdom come,
Thy will be done,
On Earth as it is in Heaven.
Give us this day
Our daily bread
And forgive us our tresspasses,
As we forgive those who trespass against us
And lead us not into temptation
But deliver us from evil.
For thine is Kingdom,
The power and the glory.
Amen

If you are at a loss for words or are feeling stuck in your communication with God, speak this prayer and you will start to feel the connection.

Reading the Bible daily can also help you find clarity and communion with God.

The passages and stories you are most drawn to are there for a reason. They speak to you on a deeper level. You can use your time and increased introspection during a fast to delve into that unconscious area and find out what they're trying to tell you.

Praying and fasting is a lot like meditating and

fasting. They share similar concepts.

Like meditation, prayer requires you to acknowledge your faults and weaknesses to begin working towards forgiveness and strength.

Prayer also teaches you to forgive those who have done you wrong. By learning to forgive you learn how to be humble and kind to those who can do you no good.

As prayer deepens your fast so to does fasting strengthen your prayer by making the spirit inside you peaceful and strong.

It calms the war that many have between their faith and their desires. By giving up on bodily desires you can focus more on your relationship with yourself and God.

However, to achieve this It is important that you fast and pray with a pure and open heart. If you're trying to achieve a selfish goal, your prayers will go unheard and your fast will end unsuccessfully.

Surprisingly, many people today think that fasting and prayer are outdated. They think that now, fasting is only reserved as a diet trend for those trying to lose weight. But fasting and prayer are just as important today as they were 100 years ago.

Fasting and prayer can even lead you to a breakthrough in life.

If there's something you've been wanting or something you've been waiting for, chances are you'll find it waiting for you at the end of your journey.

Staying Motivated

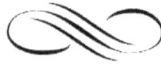

Now the big question comes into focus. How do I stay motivated during a fast?

Maybe it's been 3 days or maybe it's already been a week, but you're starting to feel tired and don't think you can keep going. Or maybe just got a huge craving that you just can't ignore.

Whatever it is, don't give in just yet!

Staying motivated is one of the biggest and hardest aspects to maintain during a fast. The first 2 weeks are especially the hardest.

This is the amount of time it usually takes for your body to adjust to receiving less food and to change from burning sugar to burning fat for energy. It's also the time when hunger and appetite will be the strongest.

Fortunately, if you can find ways to keep yourself going during that time, the days after will start to become easier and easier. Soon fasting will feel completely natural!

Tips to Stay Motivated

If you're struggling to find motivation and are at your breaking point stop for a moment and come back to this chapter. Take a moment to just go through these tips one more time.

Whether or not you choose to do one, you'll have just spent a good chunk of time not thinking about food! You've already inadvertantly distracted yourself.

Now you're probably feeling a boost of motivation. Take that feeling, pick a motivating exercise from down below and keep it going.

Find Some Inspiration

There are hundreds books and articles that talk about fasting.

Some of them are informational and some of them are personal stories, but each one of them has that bit of inspiration you need to stay motivated.

Sometimes all you really need to do is read and refresh your knowledge to remember why you started fasting in the first place. This will help you boost your confidence and rekindle your motivation.

Inspiration can also be found in other people.

You could join an online forum with people just like you who are fasting or have fasted before. Talking to them and sharing your struggles together makes you feel less alone and helps you keep each other strong.

You could also find someone to fast with. This way you have someone to spend time with, talk to and keep motivated with during your fast.

Simply having someone to share the experience can really keep you inspired to keep going.

Set Short Term Goals

If you're someone that does better with rewards then try setting some goals throughout your fast.

Give yourself a nice reward after reaching a certain length of time or even a certain weight.

For instance, you could reward yourself every 2 weeks of fasting. When that time is over treat yourself to something nice. Things like a spa day or a weekend trip are perfect for distracting yourself and making yourself feel good.

If you're going by weight, treat yourself to a shopping day when you reach your small term goal. Buying yourself nice clothes will make you look and feel better. And when you see yourself looking so good you'll only want to keep on going.

There are many different ways you can reward yourself during a fast, but you should refrain from making food your reward. This will only make it harder to stay on your fast.

Give Yourself a Cheat Day

This may seem counter-intuitive, but having a cheat day every once and a while is not so bad.

If you're craving chips have a small bag of chips. Just remember to not go overboard.

This is also the perfect time to try experimenting with healthy alternatives.

It's extremely easy to find healthy substitutes for things you're craving. Just look at any health food store and you'll see aisles fully stocked with healthy snack foods that taste good too.

You could also try making them yourself! There are thousands of recipes online that turn unhealthy snacks into a healthy alternative with just a few simple ingredient switches.

You'll have so much fun finding all these new and healthy substitutes which is perfect for motivating you towards living a healthy lifestyle. Plus, you may just learn some new cooking skills!

Visualize Your Goal

Every time you feel like quitting stop for a second and think about why you started in the first place.

Maybe you wanted to lose some weight or get that perfect beach body for the summer.

Close your eyes and picture yourself reaching that goal at the end of your fast. 9/10 that will keep you motivated.

Visualization is a very strong skill that many successful people use to stay motivated and finish what they started. By constantly visualizing yourself achieving your goal you subconciously change your attitude and actions to make it a reality.

Mood boards are great for this type of thing.

A mood board is a paper or a poster filled with all the images of things you want to achieve. They're perfect for bringing your visualizations into reality.

You could put up pictures of your ideal body, the clothes you want to fit into, the things you want to do or even the places you want to go.

Then you place that board somewhere you can see it everyday. Constantly seeing your image goals will help keep you motivated and going strong.

Focus On The Positive

Focusing on the positive is always a good idea no matter what. Whether they're big or small, positive things should always be celebrated.

Maybe you turned down dessert because it was during your fasting time or maybe you beat your craving and had a healthy snack instead.

Celebrate it! Feel good about yourself for all the little things you've accomplished.

If you feel proud of all the triumphs you achieve, big and small, you'll feel much better about yourself and what you're doing. Even when you're not feeling so good.

Your end goal doesn't have to be the only time you feel good about yourself. During your fast you'll end up achieving so many things you never thought you'd be able to.

Be Nice to Yourself

Negative thoughts and emotions are the main reason for unsuccessful fasts.

If you give into a craving or don't manage to complete your full fasting time be kind to yourself. Don't beat yourself up. You'll only make yourself feel worse which will lead you to quit.

Being hard on yourself sets a high standard that not many can fulfill. It also creates a quitting mindset that believes if you can't do it properly you shouldn't do it at all.

This is not true.

Tell yourself that it's okay you had a cheat day and ended up eating some junk food. Forgiving yourself and letting yourself know that mistakes are okay will make you feel better about trying to do better next time.

If you need to take some time to reset your mindset then take those few days off. But remember to get back to it. The longer you wait the harder it will be to return.

Keep a Journal

I touched on this lightly before and I'll mention it

again because it really does help.

Keeping a journal not only helps you keep your focus clear, it also shows you your progress.

From emotional ups and downs to physical progress, you should record it all. Write down how you feel on good days and bad days. Keep a record of your cravings and how often they come. Take pictures of your physical progress and keep track of your weight changes.

All of these are great things to remind you of how far you've progressed and why you should keep on going.

On days when you feel like quitting, go through your journal and just read through everything from the beginning. You probably won't want to give up when you see just how much you've gone through and everything you've managed to accomplish.

Spend Time with Like Minded People

Many people who fast tend to fast alone.

It's also very common for friends and family to be slightly unsupportive which can really hinder your progress. Whether they mean to be or not, if they've never done a fast, they don't understand what you're going through.

They'll probably invite you out to eat or offer you food because they've forgotten your fasting. When you have to refuse and/or constantly explain why you're fasting this can wear you down and make you feel left out.

This is why it's important to spend time with people who have done a fast or are doing a fast.

They understand what you're going through and can give you the support you need to stay motivated.

Finding people that can go along with your fast and help you make healthy choices is extremely beneficial for achieving fasting success. It also makes it 100x easier.

At the very least try to surround yourself with positive and encouraging people that will motivate you and keep you believing in your own strength.

Affirmations

Affirmations are another strong way to keep yourself motivated during your fast.

Everything you think and say to yourself is an affirmation. They can be positive or negative, but in today's world many people only practice negative affirmations.

Have you ever told you self you don't deserve something good or that you're not worth it? Have you ever put yourself down by calling yourself ugly, stupid or fat?

These are negative affirmations.

They are extremely harmful to your mind, body and spirit because they help shape your reality.

If you believe you don't deserve good things then good things won't happen to you. If you believe you're ugly then all you'll see in the mirror is someone ugly.

Toxic negative emotions and thoughts like these cause a lot of pain and suffering when they don't need to.

It's time to start practicing positive and self-empowering affirmations. During a fast is the best time to start. You're cleansing your body of harmful toxins so you should also cleanse your mind and spirit.

By repeating positive affirmations to yourself daily you can keep yourself motivated and empowered.

These affirmations can be as simple as, "You can do it," to more complex statements that are tailored specifically to you.

Affirmations can also help you reach a desired goal.

People often find when they repeat things like, "I'm going to get...," or "I deserve..." they end up getting it. This is because they are constantly reminding themselves and reaffirming their inner positivity. Therefore they unconsciously do things that will result in them getting what they want.

Affirmations are powerful tools to not only help you stay motivated during your fast but to bring into your daily life.

You will never become truly happy or satisfied until you can create your own reality. Practicing positive affirmations will help you voice your desires and bring them into your life.

Not only will you be able to control your life and get it where you want to go, you will also be less afraid and less doubtful of the things you can achieve.

Here are some powerful affirmations to get you started. You should repeat these to yourself daily.

"I am in complete control of my body during this fast."

"My body is cleansing and purifying itself during this fast."

"Every hour that I fast I become healthier, happier and have more energy and strength."

"I am using an ancient tradition, that my ancestors have used before me, to cleanse and purify my mind and body."

"I am strong and determined. Nothing can stop me from finishing my fast, not even my hunger pains."

"When I finish this fast I will have the healthy body I've always wanted."

You might feel strange when you first voice these affirmations, but that's only because your brain is not used to being so positive. That's why it's important to practice.

Daily repetitions of positive affirmations will slowly start to change your brain chemistry. It will rewire itself to start focusing only on the positive bringing happiness and joy into your life.

But saying affirmations along is not enough. You must also believe them. You must use these affirmations as instructions for your whole body to carry out. If you don't believe them then you'll just be repeating useless words to yourself.

These affirmations are true and they will work.

The Ketogenic Diet

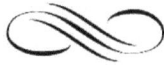

You may have heard about the Ketogenic Diet before. It's gaining popularity as a new food plan that can help people shed their stubborn body fat. But does it actually work and how?

In 1921, three compounds were discovered in the body. They became known as ketone bodies.

These ketone bodies were found to be essential for promoting detoxification and weight loss as well as being a cure for many other diseases, such as epilepsy.

However, these ketone bodies were only found in the livers of healthy patients who ate low-carbohydrate and high-fat diets. This led to the creation of the Ketogenic Diet.

This diet essentially restricts your intake of carbohydrates while relying heavily on protein and fat for energy. This puts your body into a state of ketosis. During this state your body breaks down fat and produces ketone bodies that fuel your body and brain.

This is the same thing that happens when you fast for extended periods of time. So yes, the Keto Diet actually works.

It also makes it the perfect plan for you to follow

when you've decided to break your fast. Your body remains in the same state as if you were fasting, but you're allowed to eat normally.

Well, almost normally.

You won't have to go through periods of time without eating, but you will have to watch what you eat. Foods you consume must be low in carbohydrates and high in healthy fats.

So what exactly is a carbohydrate?

It's a nutrient that provides energy for the body and brain.

Then shouldn't it be good for you?

Yes and no.

It is an essential ingredient to creating energy, but the problem is how much of it you're putting in your body.

Many people eat far above their daily need of carbohydrates. Those excess carbs are then stored for later use as fat.

The Ketogenic Diet doesn't restrict your carb intake completely, it just significantly reduces it.

That way you end up sustaining yourself with moderate amounts of protein and large amounts of fat. Your body then burns that fat for energy and you remain in ketosis.

Although this diet is extremely effective at causing weight loss, it isn't recommended for everyone. For anyone with a medical condition such as Type II Diabetes or obesity, make sure you consult your doctor before starting.

The Ketogenic Diet is a safe diet and should be able to done indefinitely, however there are no conclusive reports on if it will continue working for long periods of time. Remember to stop the diet if you start to feel unwell or any problems begin to arise.

What To Expect

There are several things you can plan to expect for when you start the Ketogenic Diet.

If you are a carb lover, then prepare yourself. Many people don't realize how many carbs are in certain foods.

Typically people think of carbs as bread and pasta, which is true.

However, high amounts of carbs are also found in rice, fruit, beans, starchy vegetables like potatoes, soda, candy and beer. Just to name a few.

During this diet you will have to restrict carb intake to about 20-50 grams a day. The less the better.

An example of this amount for one day would include a small portion of yogurt, an apple and a medium sized potato.

If you can power through this lack of carbohydrates then you can expect to see some significant health changes.

For one, lowering your carbohydrate intake leads to increased weight loss. This is because it rids your body of excess water, lowers your insulin levels and even reduces your appetite.

This means losing weight without even having to ever feel hungry.

You will also lose most of that fat from around your stomach area. This is one of the hardest places people find to lose weight.

It has to do with the type of fat that's stored in this area, visceral fat. This type of fat stores itself around your organs causing inflammation, insulin resistance and slower metabolism.

But studies have shown that lowering your carbohydrate intake helps with destroying this stubborn fat and drastically reducing the chance of getting Type 2 diabetes or heart disease.

Following the Keto diet will also lower your triglyceride count and increases the levels of good cholesterol. This means less fat circulating in the bloodstream and a lower risk of getting heart disease.

Another benefit you can receive from eating a low carbohydrate diet is found in your brain. Studies have shown that when your brain burns ketone bodies instead of sugar it can help alleviate and help prevent several brain disorders, like epilepsy, Alzheimer's and Parkinson's.

This diet has also been found to be beneficial against certain cancers, Alzheimer's and other degenerative diseases.

The Keto Diet will change the way you look at food, but it will also give you the healthy body you desire. Plus, there are many delicious foods that you can still eat that are low in carbs.

These include natural fats like olive oil and butter, seafood, meat, eggs, cheese and non-starchy vegetables like peppers, broccoli, cucumber and so on.

Generally, you want to be eating around 15-25% protein and 75% fat.

You don't want to eat too much protein because if you do it will be converted into glucose and stored as fat in your body. Something you don't want, since your ultimate goal is to burn fat.

The Keto Flu

Like any diet that restricts food, you're going to experience some side effects.

After a few days on the Ketogenic Diet you may start feeling tired, having headaches or have a hard time concentrating. This is normal and is commonly referred to as the Keto Flu.

The reason it's referred to as the Keto Flu is because many of the symptoms mimic an actual flu.

Don't worry, it's not actually a flu and it usually only lasts for 3-5 days. However, depending on your body type and how healthy you already are the time could vary and so could the symptom's strength.

Some of these symptoms include fatigue, dizziness, lightheadedness, headaches, lack of motivation, nausea and sugar cravings.

The reason for these symptoms is because your body is starting to transition from using sugar to using fat as energy.

This drastic reduction in carbohydrates results in a drop in insulin levels which takes your brain and organs sometime to get used to.

Think of carbohydrates (especially sugar) like a drug that you've been giving to yourself everyday. Now all of a sudden you're not taking that drug anymore. Like cigarettes, or cocaine or anything else highly addictive, you're going to go through some serious withdrawal symptoms.

If you've been fasting before going on this diet you should be past this stage and therefore will most likely not get the Keto Flu.

However, if you've taken a break between your fast and this diet, you may still experience some symptoms, depending on how much time has passed.

You may also experience these symptoms if you have been eating a high amount of carbs during your feast days.

The good news is there are some really simple cures to help lessen the symptoms and possibly stop them completely.

Curing the Keto Flu

Every person is different and so are their reactions to the Keto Flu.

Many report having mild to no symptoms at all, while others find they're unable to function for several days. However, the Keto Flu doesn't have to be completely unbearable.

Here are some things you can do to help drastically alleviate your symptoms.

Increase Salt and Water Intake

One of the primary reasons people get the Keto Flu is because of water and sodium loss.

When insulin levels drop it causes the body to excrete more sodium in your urine. This can easily be remedied by drinking more water and salt.

Mix half a teaspoon of salt into a glass of water and drink it whenever you feel a headache or any dizziness coming on. It should relieve your symptoms in 15-30 minutes.

If you can't handle the salty water you can also drink some consommé, bouillon soup or bone broth. There is enough salt in any of those to combat your sodium loss and they taste good too.

In general, you should always make sure you're drinking enough water. Especially during the Keto Diet because you will be losing a lot of fluids that must be replaced.

A good rule of thumb is 3 liters minimum every day for at least the 1st week of the diet.

However, the larger you are the more water you should be drinking.

Eat More Fat

Generally, increasing water and salt intake should cure most Keto Flu symptoms. However, if that still doesn't work, try adding more fat to your diet.

There's a lot of misinformation on fat today that has lead people to believe eating fat equals gaining fat. So people try to stay away from all things high in fat.

But in reality if you eat a lot of carbohydrates and not enough fat, your body will go into starvation mode and cling onto any fat in your body. Which is why most people struggle with losing weight.

When you're starting out with the Keto Diet you may be afraid to eat a lot of fat, but it's essential.

You should be eating enough fat that you don't feel

hungry after your meal. In fact, you should be able to go several hours after without feeling any hunger.

Once your body gets used to burning fat instead of sugar then you can start to cut back on your fat intake.

Just remember that fat doesn't mean protein. Later on I'll talk about the difference and give you some examples of healthy fats and proteins you can eat as well as how much of each you should be eating.

Take It Slow

If neither of the two previous options has given you any relief then you may just need to take it slow.

Everybody adapts at different rates to new things and your body may just not be ready.

You might want to try eating more carbohydrates than is required, while still keeping it to a minimum.

Start by increasing your carb intake to 75-100 grams. If you start to feel better then stick with that for a few weeks.

Once you feel ready, lower that intake to 50 grams and eventually see if you can get back down to 20 grams.

Eating more carbohydrates will slow down your weight loss and overall health improvements, but it will be easier on your mind and motivation. You will still end up reaping the Keto Diet benefits, just at a slower pace.

Slow Down on Exercise

Many people report feeling like they have more energy and strength after being on the Keto Diet, which is true. However, exercising too much can cause you to get some of the Keto Flu symptoms, especially if you do it early on.

During the first week of the Keto Diet, your physical performance will decrease due to the reduction in carbohydrates. Even professional athletes that switch to the Keto Diet experience this.

This lasts for different amounts of time, but generally around the fourth week, people start to feel better than ever.

Doing light exercises like walking, stretching and yoga are a good way to keep you active without overdoing it. It can even help reduce some of the symptoms.

But if you start to feel too burnt out then take a break from any exercise. When you're feeling better then you can begin to work your way up to more increased physical activity.

Don't Overthink It

Because of the nature of this diet many people tend to think they're overeating and that they won't lose any weight.

They start to count calories and restrict their food

intake based on that.

Counting calories or starving yourself is not how the Keto Diet works and it's not the way to lose weight or enter ketosis.

Doing this can actually aggravate your Keto Flu symptoms.

If you're worried about how much your eating, stop. Once your body transitions completely and enters ketosis your appetite will most likely decrease and you'll naturally start eating less.

During the start of your Keto Diet you should actually be eating as much of the foods you're allowed to eat until you're no longer hungry.

If you get cravings, that's fine. Have a healthy Keto snack.

Just remember to eat slowly and pay attention to your body so you don't end up overfilling yourself.

15 Healthy Foods to Eat on a Keto Diet

You may think that by restricting your diet to only high-fat, medium-protein foods, you'll be limited to only a few tasty foods. Think again!

There are many delicious and nutritious foods you can eat while still staying below the carbohydrate intake. Here is a list of my 15 favorite foods to eat on a Keto Diet and why they're so good for you.

Seafood

Seafood is a great option because it's filling and full of lots of healthy nutrients.

Both fish and shellfish are low in carbohydrates and high in fat. Plus, they're packed with Omega-3's, B vitamins and potassium. All things which contribute to healthy skin, hair and nails.

Omega-3's in particular have also been found to lower insulin levels and increase insulin sensitivity in obese people and those with diabetes.

It is extremely healthy for you and you should try to eat some form of seafood at least twice a week.

While most fish and shellfish are low in carbs some are higher than others, which is important to factor into your daily intake.

Here's an example of the carb count for some popular seafood items.

Clams contain 5 grams of carbs, octopus 4 grams, mussels 7 grams, oysters 4 grams and salmon and crab both have 0 grams.

Meat and Poultry

Meat makes up a good portion of the Keto Diet, however it should not be the main focus.

Although meat does have fat it consists primarily of protein and only a moderate amount of protein should be consumed.

If you eat too much protein on the Keto Diet it will eventually get turned into sugar and stored as fat. This will take your body out of ketosis and you may end up putting on weight rather than losing it.

This doesn't mean you can't consume any meat. Eating the right kinds of meat and in the correct amounts is perfectly fine and recommended.

Meat contains many nutrients, B vitamins and other minerals like potassium and zinc which are essential for your body.

It's the type of meat that you choose which is very important.

In general, grass-fed, free range meat is always the best choice. They have higher amounts of Omega-3's, conjugated linoleic acid and other antioxidants which they get from the grass.

Lean meats like free range chicken and turkey are also good and so is fish.

Try to stay away from non-organic, factory farmed animals. This is the cheap meat that you often see on sale in supermarkets.

These animals are full of hormones and chemicals that are meant to make the grow bigger and faster.

But this means that their meat also contains those hormones and chemicals that you later absorb into your body when you eat them. This can cause all sorts of changes to your own hormonal makeup and even promote disease.

Shirataki Noodles

You may not have heard of these noodles before, but they are often referred to as the "miracle noodle."

They're made from glucomannan, a type of fiber from the root of the konjac plant.

Shirataki noodles are traditionally an Asian ingredient that is very low in calories and carbs. In fact, 97% of their makeup is water and the remaining 3% is fiber.

They move very slowly through your digestion and therefore help you feel full for longer. Studies have shown that glucomannan also helps reduce the hormone ghrelin which is responsible for creating the feeling of hunger.

This makes Shirataki noodles the perfect addition to the Keto Diet

Besides suppressing hunger, they also have many other health benefits.

They contain prebiotics which nourish the good bacteria in your gut and help prevent inflammation as well as boost your immune system. Plus, consuming them can reduce blood sugar, helping many that suffer from diabetes.

Other health benefits of shirataki noodles include lowered cholesterol, increased insulin sensitivity and constipation relief.

Shirataki noodles can be made in a variety of ways with many different vegetables and sauces. You can also substitute them for many different dishes that require wheat noodles, allowing you to still eat your favorite foods while remaining healthy.

Non-Starchy Vegetables

These types of vegetables are low in carbs, but high in beneficial nutrients like Vitamin C.

They also contain many antioxidants that prevent damage to your cells from free radicals and a lot of fiber which is essential for smooth digestion.

Plus, leafy greens like kale and spinach have been found to combat cancer and heart disease.

Another great thing is that non-starchy vegetables can be used as substitutes for higher carb foods.

For instance, cauliflower can be processed and cooked to replace rice. Zucchini can be cut so that it resembles noodles, a type of food popularly known as "zoodles." Lettuce makes a healthy and refreshing substitute for wraps or even burgers.

These substitutes help keep your carbohydrates low and are hard to distinguish from the real thing. In fact, many tend to prefer the substitute over the real thing.

The only problem that many have when eating vegetables is their flavor. If you're used to eating very processed foods vegetables can end up tasting really bland.

Because of this people tend to add high amounts of salt or heavy amounts of sauce.

Adding sauce is fine if it's a small amount or if its homemade. Many premade sauces or dressings have lots of added sugar which you should not consume.

Olives

An olive a day keeps the doctor away.

That may not be the correct saying but it should be because olives have many health benefits that keep you living longer and stronger.

They are very low in carbohydrates and have a surprising amount of fat. 11-15% of their makeup is fat.

74% of that fat contains one particular antioxidant that is very important, oleuropein or oleic acid.

Oleic acid is extremely beneficial because of its anti inflammatory properties that protect cells from damage and disease. It also helps lower blood pressure, prevent bone loss and it may even fight cancer.

Olives make for a delicious snack or as a tasty addition to any meal.

Just make sure to get good olives preserved in oil.

Precut olives that are found in cans tend to have other preservatives added to them that render them useless in terms of health.

Avocados

Avocados are probably the best food you can eat on a Keto Diet because of their high fat content.

They're packed full of essential vitamins and minerals.

One of these important mineral, that many people are significantly lacking, is potassium which is essential for balancing sodium and keeping blood pressure low. It can also help prevent heart disease, stroke and kidney failure.

Surprisingly avocados even have more potassium than bananas. In fact, a 100 gram serving of avocados contains 14% of the recommended daily intake while bananas only have 10%.

It's possible that potassium can help reduce Keto Flu symptoms and make the transition into the Keto Diet easier.

Avocados are very filling and can help curb appetite, especially during the first few weeks of the diet.

This simple food is incredibly versatile and super delicious. You can eat them plain, sprinkled with some salt, add them to a salad or even turn them into a dessert smoothie.

Eggs

Like avocados, eggs are also extremely healthy and versatile.

It's the perfect food for a Keto Diet because they contain only 1 gram of carbs, less than 6 grams of protein and 11 grams of fat.

They've also been shown to trigger specific hormones related to feeling full. So if you eat a lot of eggs, chances are you'll feel less hunger, less often.

Many diets specify only eating certain parts of the egg, but it's important that you eat all of it. The yolks especially have many nutrients and antioxidants that are great for eye health.

The only reason people tend to avoid the yolk is because they are high in cholesterol.

However, this doesn't contribute to raising blood pressure. In fact, studies have shown that egg yolks may actually help regulate blood pressure and lower the risk of heart disease.

Eggs are also rich sources of betaine and choline, two nutrients that help reduce the risk of heart disease.

They are also important for pregnant women who are breastfeeding. Studies have shown that betaine and choline are extremely important for brain development in infants.

There are a great variety of ways you can cook and

eat eggs but there are also several different eggs that you can eat. Aside from your standard chicken egg, quail eggs and duck eggs are just as delicious and nutritious.

It's important that you buy organic free-range eggs to get the most nutrition and to stay away from dangerous hormones and chemicals.

Cheese

Many people don't think it, but cheese is actually a very healthy and nutritious thing to eat.

The other great thing about cheese is, there are hundreds of options to choose from, all of which are relatively low in carbs and high in fat.

Perfect for the Keto Diet.

Cheese contains something called conjugated linoleic acid which has been shown to increase fat loss and reduce body weight. It also protects your heart and may protect you from cancer.

If you're looking to build muscle, studies have shown that cheese may prevent muscle loss and increase muscle strength. This is due to all of the calcium, protein and B12 vitamins found in cheese.

Although cheese is high in saturated fat this shouldn't negatively affect your health if you eat it in moderate amounts and if your diet is not high in other saturated fats.

You should also opt to eat healthier cheeses. Heavily

processed cheese, like cheese sticks and Cheez-Wiz are full of sugar and other dangerous ingredients.

Try to buy cheese from the deli counter rather than from the refrigerated aisles. The deli counter often has healthier varieties of cheese, plus you can purchase them in smaller amounts.

Greek Yogurt

There's a reason Mediterraneans are known for being healthy and beautiful. It's because of all the yogurt they eat.

The difference between Greek yogurt and regular yogurt is the process it goes through when it's made.

Greek yogurt has an extra step that involves straining out the whey. This whey is what contains lactose and makes other yogurts more liquid.

By removing the lactose Greek yogurt becomes creamier and essentially healthier because it contains less sugar.

It does have a rather high carb and protein count, but its significant health benefits outweigh the excess which is why I've included it on this list.

It's full of probiotics which are great for maintaining good bacteria in your stomach and intestines. Those bacteria are what help you digest and detox properly so that you don't become backed up or full of toxins.

Eating Greek yogurt also contributes to lower blood

pressure, stronger bones, increased muscle mass and increased metabolism.

It has also been shown to help reduce appetite and the feeling of hunger.

So, if you're feeling snacky you can reach for a small thing of yogurt to satisfy your cravings. Make it even tastier with some nuts, fruits and/or spices.

Butter and Cream

Many people try to stay away from butter and cream because of their high fat content. But they are actually perfectly healthy foods that contain high amounts of good fats.

Because they are high in saturated fats many believed this was the cause of heart disease and other related illnesses.

However studies have shown that saturated fats are not linked to heart disease, as was previously thought. In fact, it there may be a link between moderate consumption of saturated fats and the reduced risk of heart disease and strokes.

They also contain many powerful antioxidants that boost the immune system and promote cell growth and repair.

One compound found in butter and cream, glycosphingolipids, has actually been found to reduce gastrointestinal disease by helping to build up the mucus layer that lines your stomach and intestines. This makes you more resistant to bacterial infections and inflammation.

Butter and cream also contain lauric acid, which is found in other healthy fats and is a significant contributing factor towards weight loss.

So the next time you reach for some butter remember that you're contributing to healthier bones, healthier guts and a healthier body.

Coconut Oil

Of all the oils you can consume, coconut oil is the best. It has unique properties that are specific onto itself.

First off, it is a medium-chain triglyceride which means it is directly absorbed by the liver and converted into ketones. So, rather than being stored in the body as fat like most oils, it is used directly as energy.

This is perfect for getting into and remaining in ketosis.

In fact, studies have shown coconut oil increases the number of ketones present in people with Alzheimer's and other brain or nervous system disorders helping to alleviate some of their symptoms.

Lauric acid, a long chain fat, present in coconut oil also helps the body remain in ketosis and kills of any harmful microorganisms like Staphylococcus and Candida Albicans.

This immediate of production of ketones has also been found to help with seizures and epilepsy.

By simply switching to coconut oil or using it daily in your meals, you can lose inches off your waist and protect yourself from many harmful diseases. All without adding any other dietary changes.

Remember to only buy organic, unprocessed coconut oil. It should smell like coconuts when you open it. Anything else is heated and overly processed rendering it useful in terms of health benefits.

Olive Oil

Olive oil is also another great source of fat that has many health benefits.

Good unprocessed olive oil is high in oleic acid which is a monounsaturated fat. These fats have been found to reduce inflammation and decrease the risk of heart disease along with many other diseases like diabetes, Alzheimer's and arthritis.

If you are taking heart disease medication, studies have shown that by adding olive oil to your diet you can reduce your need for that medication by 48%.

Olive oil is also high in antioxidants like phenol. These reduce inflammation in your arteries, promoting good heart health and good working arteries.

It's pure fat and therefore perfect for the Keto Diet.

You can add it to any meal. However, it isn't very

stable at high temperatures so only use it when cooking with low heat or by adding it to already cooked foods.

To know if you're buying good olive oil there are some general rules you should go by.

The label should always say Extra Virgin Olive Oil and it should be in a dark colored glass bottle.

If it's in a plastic bottle, it doesn't necessarily mean it's bad, it just means it won't store for as long.

Any oil that says reduced fat or light is not good oil.

Nuts and Seeds

Nuts and seeds make for fantastic additions to meals or to be used as snacks. Many of them are high in fat and low in carbs.

They're also packed with fiber leading you to feel full for longer.

Eating nuts and seeds frequently has been shown to reduce the risk of cancer, heart disease, depression and many others. In fact, eating just an ounce of nuts 4-5 times a week has been shown to protect against coronary artery disease.

Each nut and seed also has different benefits.

For example, pistachios, peanuts, pumpkin seeds and sunflower seeds have mono and polyunsaturated fats which help fight inflammation and keep cells healthy.

Almonds, hazelnuts, pecans and walnuts have many

antioxidants that help reduce the risk of heart disease.

Their carbohydrate count is also varied between them, although many of them have a very low count.

For example, almonds contain 3 grams of carbs, cashews 8 grams, macadamias 2 grams, pecans 1 gram, pistachios 5 grams, walnuts 2 grams, chia seeds 1 gram and flax seeds 0 grams.

It's important that you eat a variety of both nuts and seeds to get the most benefits out of all of them.

You should also try to purchase ones that have no added salt or sugar.

Berries

Many fruits are actually very high in carbs and therefore can't be eaten on a Keto Diet. However, berries are the exception.

All berries are good to eat on the Keto Diet, but raspberries and blackberries are especially beneficial. This is because of the amount of fiber they contain. They actually contain more fiber than carbohydrates.

Berries are also high in antioxidants that have been shown to fight inflammation, repair damaged cells and protect against many diseases.

They also lower blood pressure and increase insulin sensitivity. One study showed that consuming a blueberry smoothie twice a week drastically improved insulin sensitivity in obese people and those with diabetes.

Aside from that berries are also a beauty booster because they contain ellagic acid. This acid helps fight free radicals and block the growth of enzymes that break down collagen.

Adding some to your diet will not only improve your health and protect you from disease, it will also keep your skin young and healthy looking.

They can be added to many foods, like a fresh salad, eaten as a snack or even eaten as a dessert when you're craving some sweetness in our diet.

Dark Chocolate and Cocoa Powder

If you thought you couldn't eat any dessert on the Ketogenic diet, think again.

Dark chocolate and cocoa powder are actually full of many antioxidants that keep your heart and body healthy.

In fact, cocoa has actually been nicknamed the "super fruit" because it contains the same amount of healthy antioxidants as many other superfruits, like acai berries.

Dark chocolate is especially healthy because it contains compounds called flavanols which contribute to lower blood pressure and help clear your arteries from blockages.

Eating dark chocolate has also been shown to lower

bad cholesterol and increase good cholesterol. The many antioxidants it contains enter into the bloodstream and help protect the lipoproteins from oxidation damage.

Like berries, dark chocolate also keeps your skin healthy and youthful. The flavanols found in the chocolate protect your skin from sun damage, improve blood flow and increase skin hydration and density.

It is important that you eat the right types of chocolate. You should only be consuming dark chocolate that is 70% cocoa or more.

This is because dark chocolate has more nutrients and less sugar than chocolate with less cocoa. Dark chocolate is also extremely strong tasting which will prevent you from eating too much of it.

Creating a Ketogenic Meal Plan

Creating a meal plan is one of the easiest ways to help you stick to your diet and make sure you're eating the correct amount of foods.

I've mentioned before that around 60-80% of your food should be fats, around 15-25% should be from protein and 4-10% from carbs.

It's extremely important you follow these amounts because it's very easy for you body to get out of ketosis. It's as simple as eating an extra serving of fruit and your body starts burning sugar instead of fat.

To make it easier I've created an easy to follow

list that comprises all the foods you can eat on a Keto diet.

The first is oils and fats. These should make up most of your diet and can easily be added to any meal.

Oils and fats that are the healthiest and should be eaten regularly include olive oil, coconut oil, avocado oil, butter, heavy cream, cheese, plain yogurt and cottage cheese.

There are some other oils you may be familiar with but should be used sparingly. These include sunflower oil, safflower oil, corn oil and peanut oil.

You should never eat margarine or anything with trans fats.

The second category of foods is protein.

Consuming protein should only be done in moderate amounts and should not be the bulk of your meal.

Seafood especially has amazing benefits because of their Omega-3's. Try to consume at least 2 servings of seafood a week.

Typically your meal should consist of a small portion or protein that can include grass fed beef, fish, certain shellfish like crab or shrimp, dark meat chicken or turkey and eggs.

You may eat bacon or low fat proteins like skinless chicken or mussels, but only very rarely.

Foods like cold cuts with added sugar, meat with

sugar marinades or breaded meat like chicken nuggets should never be consumed.

Always remember to read the nutrition labels on food you are buying to check if it has added sugars.

Fruits and vegetables are make up the third food group and are great options to add to your diet. In fact, the bulk of all your meals should be mostly vegetables.

Certain vegetables can even be used as substitutes for high-carb foods. For instance, cauliflower can be ground and cooked to be used as rice.

Some fruits and vegetables that you can eat regularly include avocados, leafy greens like spinach lettuce and kale, celery, asparagus, olives, berries and dark chocolate.

Because of their high carb count you should only eat leeks, spaghetti squash and eggplant very rarely.

You should never eat potatoes, corn or raisins. They are high in carbs and sugar.

The last category of foods is nuts and seeds.

These are very healthy options to add to your meals or can also be used as a great snack. Many of them contain lots of healthy fats!

Some examples of healthy nuts and seeds are walnuts, almonds, flax seeds and chia seeds. These can be eaten regularly throughout the day or in meals.

You may also sometimes eat unsweetened nut

butters, cashew and pistachios.

However, you should never eat any sweetened nuts or seeds like trail mix with dried fruit, sweetened peanut butter or any other sweetened nut butter and chocolate covered nuts.

A Life After Fasting

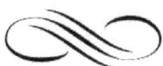

Now you know everything there is to know about intermittent fasting.

You're all hyped up and ready to get started right? Fantastic.

But what happens when you've safely broken and successfully completed your fast? How do you continue to keep the weight off and maintain a healthy lifestyle?

Well, hopefully during your fast you've already picked up some healthy habits along the way. It's almost impossible to maintain a fast while eating unhealthy foods and living an inactive lifestyle.

But the real challenge comes by trying to stop yourself from falling back into old destructive habits.

One of the keys to actually sticking with your new healthy lifestyle is fasting regularly.

This doesn't have to mean everyday for the rest of your life. But it does mean at least twice a year or possibly even more.

If you can actively sustain an intermittent fast everyday for the rest of your life then by all means do it. You could even increase your fasting power by doing a

24 or more hour fast several times during the year.

Not only does this keep your body in shape and in a fat burning state, it also actively reminds you what it feels like to be healthy and what you need to do to achieve this state.

However, if you can't or don't want to keep fasting everyday then there are some things you need to do during your break to stay healthy and to keep the weight off.

First off, it's important that you remain engaged in a healthy lifestyle. This means eating wholesome, nutritious food and staying active.

You can't return to eating junk food and sitting on your couch and expect to maintain your healthy fasted body.

Secondly, if you want to achieve your body's ultimate health and energy power, you must think of fasting as an ongoing cycle. Each time you start a fast you should be healthier than the time before.

This will make the fasting process easier and it will also help your body purge itself of toxins on a deeper level. Just when you think you've gone as far as you can with fasting you'll find there's always something new to be learned and experienced.

In turn, regular fasting will give you some healthy habits.

One habit will be an increased ability and desire to

eat healthier foods. Once you've completed a fast successfully you should be able to eat at least 40% more raw fruits and vegetables. What's more, you'll actually want to eat those foods and possibly even start to crave them.

This may come as a surprise but your body actually does want to eat healthy foods. It's just be dulled over the years with excessive fats, salts and sugars. But clearing it out, through fasting, will let your cravings for good nutrition become heard again.

It won't happen overnight, nor will it happen after your first fast. Resetting your body back to its pure state will be slow and difficult at first and it will take time for you body to get used to eating healthy again.

But you will get there!   And over time it will only get easier.

The most important thing you need to remember right now is to listen to your body. There are so many different opinions on nutrition and health. Some say to eat high fat, low carbs. Some say eat low fat, high carbs. Some say vegetarian is better while others say vegan is the healthiest way to eat.

It's hard to know who's right and in reality, they're all a little bit right. Because the real key is eating in balance.

You can eat protein. You can eat fat. You can even eat sugar.

As long as it's balanced with all the other foods you're eating.

If you're looking for an easy way to health or for me to tell you exactly what to eat to lose weight then you're in the wrong place. Health and eating are both completely personal because each body is unique.

What might taste good for me, might taste horrible to you. What might fuel me up with tons of energy, might make you feel tired and sick. What I might think is the most nutritious food, you might be allergic to.

The only thing I can do is put you on the right path to long lasting health.

That starts with fasting, eating healthy and staying active.

As long as you continue to participate in those three things, you should feel younger and more energetic than ever.

It was always Mother Nature's intention for us to have healthy bodies. It was just our human arrogance that believed it could break certain laws and still retain its health. But in the end we are the ones suffering.

It is entirely possible for you to live without chronic illness, without bodily injury and without even so much as a sniffle. The only price you have to pay is giving up artificiality.

Say no to junk food. Say no to processed food. Say no to an lazy lifestyle.

By learning to say no you will be able to say yes to so many things that will end up keeping you happy and fulfilled.

If you've ever wanted to live life to its fullest then learning to say no is the first step.

Be the creator of your own life.

Don't let others dictate your life for you.

Set your standard for healthy living and carry it out. And whenever you're in doubt, turn to Mother Nature for advice.

Everything she provides is there for a reason.

Use this book as a guide to help you on your journey to a better and brighter future of living. It will provide advice and motivation whenever you're in need.

Always remember that you are stronger than you think and that your health, happiness and future are in your hands only.

Common Questions

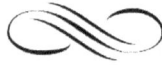

In this short chapter I'll being answering some of the most common questions I hear on intermittent fasting.

All of these questions have been discussed in detail in previous chapters. This section is just to be used as a reference for quick information.

Isn't intermittent fasting basically starving yourself? Won't this slow down your metabolism and make losing weight harder?

This is one of the most common misconceptions about fasting. It is not starvation!

Starvation is involuntary whereas fasting is voluntary.

To put it even more simply, starvation is when you get trapped somewhere without food or water. Fasting is when you know you can eat, but choose not to.

In fact, the only thing different between fasting and eating normally is the time in which you do it. You're not restricting calories nor are you giving up food completely.

There are some fasting methods that do have you go several days without food, but at the end you always return to eating.

It actually takes quite a long time for your body to enter into starvation mode. The problem is many people are used to eating and so they end up feeling like they're starving when they miss a meal.

Of course, this also depends on how much you weigh at the start of your fast, but it's safe to say you won't end up starving during an intermittent fast.

In fact, the world record for fasting was 382 days without food at all. And the person who completed this fast was perfectly healthy at the end.

Fasting also won't slow down your metabolism, like many people think it will.

As long as you're eating enough calories during your feasting time and doing some form of exercise your metabolism should remain the same and can even increase.

If you start to restrict your caloric intake when you eat (as many do) then your metabolism will start to slow as it tries to preserve the fat it does have.

Keeping a balance between eating, fasting and exercising will allow you to lose the most weight and overall body fat in a shorter amount of time.

Is it safe for anyone to fast? Or should only really healthy people be doing it?

It is perfectly safe for anyone to do intermittent

fasting.

If you're old, young, healthy, overweight and even suffering from a disease you should be able to still fast.

However, to be on the safe side it's important you get your doctor's consent before you start if you aren't perfectly healthy to begin with.

That being said, fasting can actually help a lot of people that are suffering from some sort of illness.

Not only does it boost your immune system, it also strengthens your brain. Studies have shown that intermittent fasting can help prevent many common diseases like Type II diabetes, heart disease, stroke, Alzheimer's, Parkinson's and even cancer.

The only people who don't really need to fast are children. They are growing and need a lot of food to help give their body the nourishment it needs.

It's just important that they eat the right foods and don't overeat.

If a child is suffering from obesity they may benefit from some intermittent fasting, however, it can be just as helpful to reduce the amount of sugar and fats they're consuming.

What if I'm extremely skinny, won't it be bad for me to fast?

Leaner people tend to think that fasting is just for those who want to lose weight, but fasting is also a great way to gain weight.

In terms of muscle mass that is.

You shouldn't do intermittent fasting if you are very underweight or suffering from some type of eating disorder. If you want to try it consult with your doctor first to make sure it won't hurt you.

Now, if you are a healthy person but just have a very skinny body type then you could benefit from doing a fast.

Just because you're skinny doesn't mean your body isn't using sugar as energy. It also doesn't mean that you don't have any fat to burn.

Fat is stored in many places of the body, including muscle. And by getting your body to burn that fat you could increase your muscle building power.

In fact, the problem many skinny people have when trying to gain muscle is that they're not burning fat. So, if you've ever wanted to build your muscle mass or add some definition to your thin frame then do a fast.

The only thing you'll need to keep in mind is how much you're eating during your feasting window. To burn fat and build muscle you'll need to be consuming a lot of calories most of which are from fat. This way your body will always have an endless amount of fat to burn for energy.

When do I start counting my 16 hours of fasting? By the time I eat my last meal or after I finish eating

it?

You fasting window is a period of time that you do not eat anything.

So your fasting time would start when you finish your last meal. For example, if you start your last meal at 6pm and finish it by 7pm then your fasting time would start at 7pm.

Alternatively you would not start eating until after 11am.

Can women and men follow the same fasting protocols or should they each do something different?

Yes, it's true. Men and women are not same. At least bodywise.

Generally, women are smaller than men, which means they don't need to fast as long as men to achieve the same benefits. It also means they don't need to eat as much food as men.

There are many women who can do 16 hour fasts or longer and feel fine, but studies have shown that they don't really need to do it for that long to achieve the same benefits.

Women are also more sensitive to hunger so it may not be as easy for them to do longer fasts than men.

If you're restricting calories during fasting time men need to have more than women. So women should restrict their calories to 500-600 while men should stick around 1000-1200 calories.

In terms of breaking a fast, men should be eating more food than women and of a different variety. Of course, both should have a healthy serving of vegetables but men also need to have more protein and fat in their diet than women.

Women should also not do an intermittent fast when they are trying to conceive or if they are currently pregnant.

During my fasting time can I drink coffee or tea? They have calories so won't that put me out of my fasting state?

Drinking coffee or tea during your fast is fine and even recommended to help with hunger. You will still remain in a fasted state as long as your drink stays under 50 calories.

If you're using premade coffee powders you should probably check the calorie count because many of them have added ingredients. However, fresh ground coffee is perfectly fine.

You could even put a little splash of milk or cream.

This may slow down your fat burning by a little, but it will also help take the edge off your hunger. Just make sure to stay away from sugar.

You should also make sure you're drinking a lot of water, especially if you're drinking coffee.

In general you want to make sure you stay hydrated throughout your fast. But coffee is a diuretic which causes you to urinate a lot and can lead to dehydration.

How often can I eat during the eating times? Is it okay if I eat a snack in between meals?

A lot of people tend to think there's only a specific amount they can eat during the eating time window. But really you can eat as much as you want.

Fasting has nothing to do with calorie restriction.

You're not limited to how much or how often you can eat, you're just limited to a specific time that you can eat.

Some people only eat 2 meals because it's easier and they don't get hungry as often. But, others like to eat several meals and snack during their eating window.

There's really no rule on this. The only thing that matters is that you do it during your 8 hour time frame.

I'm always starving by the time I get to my eating window. How can I fill myself up more so I don't break my fast too early?

Lots of people feel extreme hunger during the first couple of weeks of fasting. That's normal.

It's mainly because you're body is just used to eating a certain amount at a certain time.

However, you could also be feeling hungry because you're not eating the right types of food. If your body is missing a nutrient or vitamin this will result in you feeling some sort of discomfort.

Rather than trying to meet a specific caloric intake, like many do when fasting, focus on fulfilling your body's basic requirements.

This is done easily by eating a large variety of foods. You should be eating a lot of different vegetables and meats, with vegetables making up the bulk of your meal.

You could also eat foods high in fat, like avocados, which will help keep you feeling full for longer.

How you eat is also a determining factor in keeping hunger away.

Try eating slowly. This is better for your digestion and helps your body absorb nutrients easier.

When your body is well nourished it doesn't feel like it needs to eat as much.

Some people also find that eating smaller meals several times throughout the day helps trick their brain into feeling like it's getting a lot of food.

I have a very busy schedule during the day and don't really have time to make every meal. How can I work intermittent fasting into my routine so that I'm able to eat during the right time?

Intermittent fasting is actually one of the easiest ways to eat for people that are extremely busy. Often times those people are already participating in intermittent fasting without realizing it.

However, if you're serious about doing intermittent fasting properly while having a busy schedule it will require a lot of planning.

First, you should choose a fasting/feasting window that works best with your day.

If you have to work early you might want to start eating around lunch time. If you work later hours starting your feasting time at breakfast might be better.

It really all depends on you and which meals you really want to eat.

The second step is meal planning and preparation.

Busy people usually don't have time to prepare and cook good healthy meals. That's why so many end up eating junk food snacks or fast food.

You can save yourself from this by making your meals ahead of time. There are thousands of recipes online that are dedicated specifically to meal prep.

Depending on your schedule you can make them the day before or even make a whole week's worth of meals on the weekend. That way you don't have to worry about cooking and all your meals are ready to grab and go.

The important thing to remember is that your meals are balanced, healthy and preferably homemade. Stay away from ready-made lunches or anything frozen that you can buy in the supermarket.

Won't I lose muscle mass from fasting? How can I keep that from happening?

Generally, during the first few weeks of intermittent fasting you body will start to lose some muscle mass along with fat. This is because of the transition it goes through from burning sugar to burning fat.

However, intermittent fasting allows you to lose more weight while keeping more muscle than a normal fat busting diet would.

You will also not be as energetic during the start of your fast so your workout performance may decrease contributing to this loss in muscle mass.

Once you completely transition and regain the energy to workout your muscle mass and strength will slowly start to increase. Your performance will also increase and you'll be able to exercise for longer periods of time without getting fatigued.

The real key to keeping and building muscle mass while fasting is through strength training.

Lifting weights and doing body weight exercises will help strengthen and tone your muscles into perfect shape.

You should also be consuming a good amount of high quality protein after your workouts to feed your muscles.

A good rule to follow is 1 gram of protein for every pound of weight. So if you weigh 120 pounds, you should be eating 120 grams of protein every day.

How often should I be working out? Is there such a thing as too much?

Once your body gets past the initial stages of fasting and starts burning fat you will start to notice a significant difference in your energy levels.

How often you work out and how much you do is really up to your personal preference. Just make sure you listen to your body and don't push it to the point of injury.

If you're someone who likes to workout often then working out everyday at lower intensities might suit you. If you don't have time to workout everyday then you could exercise for shorter amounts of time at higher intensities.

Both of these options will get you the same results, but choosing one that fits your routine and body will make it easier on your mind and motivation.

Most experts recommend only doing 2-3 strength training sessions for every 7-10 days when you're doing intermittent fasting. However, if you feel you can do more without hurting yourself then that's always a possibility.

Just make sure you're doing different types of workouts each day. Don't just stick to cardio, for instance. You will get the best results if you mix and match exercises that workout your whole body in different ways.

Can I take breaks during my intermittent fast or will that ruin the whole process?

Of course you can take breaks. That's what intermittent fasting is all about.

For example, if you want to only do it on the weekdays while continuing to eat normally on weekends that's perfectly fine.

You will still reap the rewards of the fast as long as there isn't too much time between your fasts. A day or two will not ruin the process. It will just slow it down.

If you are doing longer periods of fasting, 24 hours or more, then it's actually very important that you take breaks in between.

If you are doing the 16/8 fast or another one like it, then breaks aren't that important. You could even potentially do it for the rest of your life.

However, in the beginning of any fast you may need some days to adjust and therefore taking breaks when you need it will help make the transition easier and more manageable.

Try to remember that fasting is not about pushing your body to extreme lengths. It's about getting your body to start burning fat instead of sugar. Therefore, it's not so important to force yourself to keep from eating when you start to feel extremely hungry.

www.ingramcontent.com/pod-product-compliance
Lightning Source LLC
Chambersburg PA
CBHW050735030426
42336CB00012B/1570